REPORT

Improving the Deployment of Army Health Care Professionals

An Evaluation of PROFIS

Melony E. Sorbero • Stuart S. Olmsted • Kristy Gonzalez Morganti • Rachel M. Burns Ann C. Haas • Kimberlie Biever

Prepared for the United States Army
Approved for public release; distribution unlimited

RAND ARROYO CENTER and RAND HEALTH

The research described in this report was sponsored by the Army Office of the Surgeon General. It was conducted jointly by RAND Arroyo Center and RAND Health. RAND Arroyo Center, part of the RAND Corporation, is a federally funded research and development center sponsored by the United States Army.

Library of Congress Cataloging-in-Publication Data

Sorbero, Melony E.
  Improving the deployment of Army health care professionals : an evaluation of PROFIS / Melony E. Sorbero, Stuart S. Olmsted, Kristy Gonzalez Morganti, Rachel M. Burns, Ann C. Haas, Kimberlie Biever.
    pages cm
  Includes bibliographical references.
  ISBN 978-0-8330-7804-9 (pbk. : alk. paper)
  1. United States. Army—Medical personnel. 2. United States. Army—Personnel management. I. Title.

  UH223.S63 2013
  355.3'450973—dc23

                                                                              2013008370

Published 2013 by the RAND Corporation
1776 Main Street, P.O. Box 2138, Santa Monica, CA 90407-2138
1200 South Hayes Street, Arlington, VA 22202-5050
4570 Fifth Avenue, Suite 600, Pittsburgh, PA 15213-2665
RAND URL: http://www.rand.org/
To order RAND documents or to obtain additional information, contact
Distribution Services: Telephone: (310) 451-7002;
Fax: (310) 451-6915; Email: order@rand.org

Preface

The Army Medical Department's (AMEDD's) Professional Filler System (PROFIS) was developed in 1980 to support continuous overseas contingency operations while simultaneously balancing the Army's requirement to maintain a healthy force, deploy a medical force to support military operations, and manage/meet access-to-care demands for all military health system beneficiaries. PROFIS allows health care providers to practice in a military treatment facility (MTF) when not deployed, which contributes to the maintenance of their medical and technical skills. The PROFIS Deployment System (PDS), developed in 2005, is an internal management system that is used to battle roster deploying units with the correct PROFIS personnel so that the U.S. Army Medical Command (MEDCOM) can plan proactively for deployments. Recently, there have been concerns over how PROFIS affects the medical readiness and availability of providers for training with the unit preparing to deploy.

This report describes the functionality of the Army's PROFIS in the current operating environment and assesses potential modifications or improvements to the system.[1] Using a literature review, interviews, a survey, and administrative data, this research sought to identify and understand the effect of PROFIS, and deployments more broadly, on providers and other military personnel. The study also assessed modifications and alternatives to the current PROFIS that might address the identified issues. The contents of this report will be of interest to national policymakers, MEDCOM, health care providers, MTF commanders, health care provider organizations, and others who seek to optimize the deployment of medical personnel and to understand the effects of deployments on medical personnel skills and retention in the military.

The Army Office of the Surgeon General sponsored this study. It was conducted jointly by RAND Arroyo Center and RAND Health. RAND Arroyo Center, part of the RAND Corporation, is a federally funded research and development center sponsored by the United States Army.

The Project Unique Identification Code (PUIC) for the project that produced this document is DASGP10527.

---

[1] This volume contains the main text of the report and three appendixes. Additional appendixes, which detail results from analyses of corps-specific data, the web survey, and regression analyses, are available at http://www.rand.org/pubs/technical_reports/TR1227.html.

Contents

Preface iii

Figures ix

Tables xi

Summary xiii

Acknowledgments xix

Abbreviations xxi

CHAPTER ONE

Introduction 1

Background 1

Purpose and Approach 2

How This Report Is Organized 3

CHAPTER TWO

Background 5

Factors Leading to the Development of PROFIS 5

PROFIS Overview 6

Turmoil in the System 8

Changes to Deployment Length for PROFIS Personnel During OEF/OIF 10

Deployment of Medical Personnel in Other Services 12

  Navy 12

  Air Force 13

Deployment of Medical Personnel in Selected Other Countries 14

  Differences in Health Care Systems 15

  How Services Are Provided to Armed Forces 15

  Personnel Deployed 17

  Length of Deployment 17

CHAPTER THREE

Data and Methods 19

Key-Informant Interviews.. 19

Survey 20

  Survey Items 21

  Survey Eligibility and Sampling 22

  Survey Dissemination 22

    Survey Analyses 23
Army Medical Department Resource Tasking System (ARTS) Data 29
Administrative Data 30
    Administrative Data Analyses 31

CHAPTER FOUR
Effect of and Concerns About PROFIS 35
Stakeholders and Issues 35
Equity of Deployments 36
Battalion Surgeon Positions 43
Predictability 47
Skills and Training 47
Impact on Military Treatment Facilities 51
Retention 53
Summary of Key Observations 56
    Equity 56
    Predictability 58
    Skills and Training 59
    Impact on Military Treatment Facilities 59
    Retention 59

CHAPTER FIVE
Potential Modifications to PROFIS 61
Increase the Supply of Providers Available for Deployment 63
    Limit Consecutive Assignments in Nondeployable Positions 63
    Reduce Nondeployable Profiles in Deployable Positions 64
    Improve Rewards for Deployment 65
    Delay Fellowships 65
    Shift Requirements to Increase AOCs in Demand 65
    Offer Long-Term Civilian Contracts 66
    Deploy Civilians to Combat Support Hospitals 66
Make Changes to the Battalion Surgeon Position 66
    Create a Battalion Surgeon Training Module 67
    Shorten Battalion Surgeon Deployment Length 67
    Have Interns Practice as General Medical Officers Prior to Completing Residency 68
    Use Physician Extenders as Battalion Surgeons 68
    Use Borrowed Military Manpower for Battalion Surgeons 69
Improve Predictability of PROFIS 70
    Improve Timeliness of Orders 70
    Make Changes to the Frequency and/or Timing of PDS Conference 71
    Implement Long-Term PROFIS Assignments 71
    Implement ARFORGEN Cycle for PROFIS Positions 72
    Use Borrowed Military Manpower for All Health Care Personnel 72
Reduce Impact of Deployment on Military Treatment Facilities 73
    Increase Civilian Staff at Military Treatment Facilities 73
    Implement a National Backfill Contract 74

Reduce Skills Degradation..74
    Have No Deployment in the Year Following Clinical Training.......................74
    Make a Formal Assessment of Need for Retraining Upon Redeployment............75
Improve Other Equity Issues..75
    Eliminate 90-Day Post-Stabilization Period..75
    Switch All Officer AOCs to Tier I and Manage Centrally...........................76
Summary...76

CHAPTER SIX
Conclusions and Recommendations...77
Recommendations..77
    Modifications That Could Be Implemented Individually and in the Near Term........78
    Modifications Potentially Best Implemented as an Integrated Approach..............80
Summary...81

APPENDIXES
A. PROFIS Areas of Concentration/Military Occupational Specialties,
    by PROFIS Tier and Number of Army Personnel in Each, as of December 2009.....83
B. AOCs, by Strata, Used in the Survey Sampling and Analyses.......................89
C. AOCs That Are Allowed Substitutions for the Battalion Surgeon..................95

Appendixes D–N are available online at
    http://www.rand.org/pubs/technical_reports/TR1227.html

References..97

Figures

2.1. Percentage of All Deployments of Health Care Professionals During OEF/OIF (2002–2009) Filled by PROFIS Personnel, by Corps 9

2.2. Distribution of PROFIS Deployments During OEF/OIF Across Corps (2002–2009).... 9

2.3. Changes to PROFIS/PDS During OEF/OIF 11

3.1. Conceptual Model of Deployment Experiences on Impact of PROFIS and Retention Intentions... 24

4.1. Percentage of Personnel-Time Deployed, by Corps and Quarter (PROFIS and Organic).. 37

4.2. Highest and Lowest Percentages of Personnel-Time Deployed, by Quarter (PROFIS and Organic).. 38

4.3. Number of Deployments (PROFIS and Organic) per Individual, by Corps, for Personnel in the Army in December 2009 39

4.4. Percentage of PROFIS Deployments Starting in 2009 That Were Less Than or Equal to Nine Months or Greater Than Nine Months in Duration, by Corps 42

4.5. Views of Personnel on Equity of PROFIS 42

4.6. Physicians Filling Battalion Surgeon Deployments (2002–2010) 44

4.7. Views on PROFIS Equity Among Physicians Able to Deploy as Battalion Surgeons, by Whether They Deployed as Battalion Surgeons or in Other Positions 45

4.8. Among Physicians Able to Deploy as Battalion Surgeons, the Average Length of Deployments, by Deployment Type 45

4.9. Extent to Which Physicians Able to Fill Battalion Surgeon Positions Felt Clinically Prepared When Deployed as Battalion Surgeons, Compared with Other Deployments, by Type of Specialty.. 46

4.10. Extent to Which Physicians Able to Fill Battalion Surgeon Positions Report Experiencing Skill Degradation While Deployed as Battalion Surgeons, Compared with Other Deployments, by Type of Specialty 46

4.11. Reported Timing of Notification and Orders for PROFIS Personnel Prior to Deployment 48

4.12. Satisfaction with Timing of Orders for Deployment...................................... 48

4.13. Total Number of Reclamas, by Year and Type of Request................................ 49

4.14. Impact of Deployment on Clinical and Surgical Skills 50

4.15. Impact of PROFIS Deployments on Military Treatment Facilities........................ 52

4.16. Intentions of Health Care Professionals to Remain on Active Duty After Their Current Service Obligation Ends 54

4.17. Effect of Satisfaction with Family Support on Spouses' Desire to Stay in or Leave the Army... 55

4.18. Survival Curves Describing Months Deployed Prior to End of ADSO and Percentage Staying in the Army After ADSO for Officers... 57

4.19.   Estimated Effects of Cumulative Months of Deployment on the Percentage of
        Enlisted Corps Choosing to Reenlist at the First Reenlistment Decision, Over Time.... 58

Tables

S.1. Promising Modifications to PROFIS and Their Qualitative Impacts xvi
2.1. Comparison of Health Care Systems, Physician Employment, Mandatory Military Service, and Provision of Medical Care to Military Populations for Selected Allied Countries 16
3.1. Key Issues Identified During Interviews and Data Used to Assess 21
3.2. Categories of Questions from PROFIS Survey 22
3.3. Survey Sample Size, by Strata 23
3.4. Response Rate, by Corps 24
3.5. Comparison of Responders to Nonresponders, by Corps: Rank 25
3.6. Comparison of Responders to Nonresponders, by Corps: Base Active Service Duty Years 26
3.7. Demographic Characteristics of Responders 27
3.8. Military Service Characteristics of Responders 28
4.1. Issues About PROFIS, by Stakeholder 36
4.2. Adjusted Probability of Deployment, by Demographics and Service Characteristics, with at Least One Deployment Among Active-Duty Personnel in December 2009 40
4.3. Impact of Deployment on Leadership Skills 51
4.4. Rates, Impact, and Satisfaction of Backfill, by Corps 53
4.5. Survey Respondent Retention Intentions 54
5.1. Potential Modifications to PROFIS and Their Qualitative Impacts 62
5.2. Assessment of Potential Modifications to Increase the Supply of Health Care Professionals Available for Deployment 64
5.3. Assessment of Potential Modifications That Change the Battalion Surgeon Position 67
5.4. Assessment of Potential Modifications to Improve the Predictability of PROFIS 70
5.5. Assessment of Potential Modifications to Reduce Impact of Deployments on MTFs 73
5.6. Assessment of Potential Modifications to Reduce Skills Degradation During Deployment 74
5.7. Assessment of Other Potential Modifications to Improve Equity of Deployments 75
A.1. Tier I AOCs/MOSs 83
A.2. Tier II AOCs/MOSs 85
A.3. Tier III AOCs/MOSs 87
B.1. Strata for Each Corps 89
B.2. Specific AOCs/MOSs Within Each Strata 90
C.1. Allowed Substitutions for Battalion Surgeon Positions 95

Summary

Background and Purpose

The Army Medical Department (AMEDD) has multiple missions, including to provide a medical force that supports deployed operations and to deliver health care to soldiers and retirees and their families. The AMEDD does not have enough medical personnel to simultaneously fully staff the requirements it has for both (1) deployable Table of Organization and Equipment (TOE) units, such as combat support hospitals (CSHs), that are under the command of the U.S. Army Forces Command (FORSCOM) or other commands, and (2) Table of Distribution and Allowances (TDA) units, such as military treatment facilities (MTFs), clinics, and other commands on Army bases, which are under the command of the U.S. Army Medical Command (MEDCOM). To accomplish both missions, most medical personnel are permanently assigned to TDA units and are temporarily reassigned by MEDCOM to fill or augment TOE units with additional medical personnel when these units are preparing for deployment. Upon redeployment, these personnel return to their assigned MTFs (or other assignments). MEDCOM uses a system called the Professional Filler System (PROFIS) to accomplish this. In addition, it utilizes the PROFIS Deployment System (PDS) as a selection and management system to improve the predictability and equity of PROFIS deployments in the current rotational deployment environment. It is used to fill requirements with appropriate personnel for units scheduled to deploy within the following year. PDS separates health care professionals by area of concentration (AOC), for officers, or military occupation specialty (MOS), for enlisted personnel, into tiers based on their numbers and deployment schedule, which determine whether PROFIS assignments are decided nationally (Tier I), at the regional medical commands and major subordinate commands (Tier II), or within individual MTFs (Tier III).

Although MEDCOM has been able to fill all of its PROFIS deployment requirements, AMEDD leaders are concerned that the contemporary operating environment of persistent conflict is taxing PROFIS and PDS and that the PROFIS/PDS system is not fully meeting the expectations it was designed to satisfy, such as providing soldiers and deploying units with predictability and equity among deployments. The system also potentially generates negative consequences, including dissatisfaction among health care professionals that may affect their retention, and reduced access to care at the home station when PROFIS personnel deploy.

These concerns prompted the Army Surgeon General to ask RAND Arroyo Center to study PROFIS and assess its effects on providers and on nonmedical Army personnel, determine whether the issues that led to the establishment of PROFIS still remain, and determine whether there should be an alternative to PROFIS or whether PROFIS itself needs improvement. To answer these questions, we (1) reviewed the literature and interviewed key stakeholders; (2) analyzed databases to determine which health care professionals were deployed, how often, and for how long; and (3) conducted a web-based survey of Army health care professionals. We also drew data from another RAND Arroyo Center project that was assessing the ability of MTFs to care for beneficiaries during deployments. Based on this information, we identified and assessed potential modifications to the system.

Findings

We identified four areas of concern related to PROFIS: predictability, skills and training, impact on MTFs, and equity.

Predictability

Predictability was a concern for both those who deploy as part of the system and those who interact with it. Health care professionals, who deploy as part of PROFIS, reported that notification often came very close to the time of deployment, giving them little time to prepare. The absence of official orders often exacerbated the challenge of short preparation time. Orders are necessary to carry out many of the activities that must occur before deploying personnel depart, such as arranging housing issues and storing household goods.

For those units receiving PROFIS personnel, the issue was different. Interviewees told us that the name of the PROFIS individual who was going to be deploying with the unit would often change and sometimes changed multiple times. This hampered the unit's ability to incorporate the PROFIS individual into the predeployment training so that he or she could become familiar with the unit personnel and its operating procedures.

Skills and Training

Skills and training were also issues for both health care professionals and receiving units. Health care professionals want to be well trained for the position they are filling, and they do not want their skills to degrade while deployed. Receiving units want their PROFIS fillers to have the required clinical skills, but units also need their health care professionals to have appropriate soldier skills.

Some receiving units reported that their PROFIS fillers were not as well prepared as they could have been, especially with regard to solider skills, while health care professionals reported that the 30 days of predeployment training that some of them had to participate in was not very useful. In addition, 20–30 percent of subspecialty-trained physicians who deployed as battalion surgeons reported that they were poorly prepared for the clinical duties that they were expected to perform.

Fifty percent of physicians who had deployed reported in the survey that their clinical or surgical skill decreased while deployed. Two main reasons for this were suggested during interviews. First, when deployed, physicians and other clinicians may not use the same skills as when they are working in an MTF. For example, an obstetrician rarely delivers a baby while deployed. Second, even if they are performing similar activities while deployed as they would in the MTF, they may not have enough cases to maintain their skills. Skill degradation was not universally the case; many nonphysician health care professionals reported improvement in their skills, especially their leadership skills.

Effect on Military Treatment Facilities

Health care professionals who deploy under PROFIS are typically pulled from their permanent duty stations at the MTFs. While the facilities and regional commands make efforts to replace them, this does not always occur, and the remaining staff must spread the workload across fewer personnel. In those cases where a backfill is provided, it does not always cover the entire period of the deployment. Consequently, those who remain behind have an increased workload. A secondary effect, which we were not able to establish definitively, is a perceived reduction in access to medical care for those remaining behind at the installation.

Equity

Not all health care providers deploy, and among those who do, some deploy more frequently and for longer periods than others.

We found that deployment frequency varies by medical AOC. In most AOCs, less than 10 percent of the members deployed two or more times in the 2002–2009 period. However, in some AOCs a much larger fraction of personnel have deployed more than twice. For example, over 45 percent of physician assistants, nurse anesthetists, and general surgeons have deployed two or more times. Even in these AOCs, however, there are people who have not deployed at all. This can lead to a perception that the system is not equitable, particularly among those who have deployed; this is a view that approximately 20 percent of the Nurse Corps, Medical Specialist Corps, and Medical Service Corps and a third of the Medical Corps hold. This study showed that those who feel unequally treated by PROFIS have a lower propensity to remain in the Army compared with other health care providers.

Part of the reason that more physicians view PROFIS as inequitable is the battalion surgeon position. Battalion surgeon deployments are typically longer than other physician deployments, and physicians are more likely to report skills degradation and being clinically unprepared for their deployed duties when they have deployed as a battalion surgeon.

Conclusions

Based on our analyses, we arrived at the following ten conclusions:

- PROFIS generally works. It enables the Army to deploy the required number of health care professionals with the appropriate skills, but there are areas for improvement.
- PROFIS is largely viewed as equitable, but a sizable minority view it as inequitable.
- Those who perceive it as inequitable were more likely to have deployed during Operation Enduring Freedom (OEF) or Operation Iraqi Freedom (OIF).
- Deployments differ substantially in number and length depending on the AOC of the health care professional.
- Filling the battalion surgeon position imposes additional demands on PROFIS personnel, including longer deployments and skills mismatch.
- A substantial percentage of PROFIS deployers receive notification of deployment and delivery of formal orders very late in the process.
- The PROFIS selection process involves noticeable turmoil, which reduces predictability for the PROFIS deployers and the units to which they are assigned.

- Physicians reported degradation of their clinical skills during deployment, particularly when deployed as a battalion surgeon; however, almost all perceived improvement in their leadership skills.
- PROFIS deployments result in the perception of increased workload and reduced access to medical care at the MTF from which health care professionals deploy.
- Health care professionals who have long or multiple deployments and perceive PROFIS as inequitable report a decreased propensity to remain in the military.

Modifications

We have identified 23 potential modifications to PROFIS, which are described in Chapter Five. No one modification addresses all of the issues that stakeholders raised regarding PROFIS. Indeed, some will likely have mixed effect, improving things for some stakeholders and making them worse for others. From these potential modifications, we selected 11 (Table S.1) that we view as most promising, which are discussed in Chapter Six. In Table S.1, we have distinguished between (1) those that could be done independently and quickly but with modest effect and (2) those that would have greater effect but are more difficult to implement, in part because they would require a more complex integrated approach. The modifications requiring an integrated approach are highlighted in gray in Table S.1.

Table S.1
Promising Modifications to PROFIS and Their Qualitative Impacts

Category	Potential Modification	Issues Affected
Increase the supply of health care professionals available for deployment	Limit the number of consecutive assignments to nondeployable positions (e.g., Office of the Surgeon General, Deputy Commander of Clinical Services, Deputy Commander for Nursing).	Equity; impact on MTFs; retention
	Limit the number of personnel with nondeployable profiles assigned to deployable positions. (Assign personnel with nondeployable profiles to "fenced positions" or other nondeployable positions.)	Equity; impact on MTFs; retention
	Shift the requirements for number of personnel in each AOC to increase personnel in AOCs in higher demand for deployment (e.g., increase supply of physician assistants or general surgeons).	Equity; skills and training; impact on MTFs; retention
	Offer long-term civilian contracts for Army-trained subspecialists (all corps).	Equity; skills and training; impact on MTFs; retention
Change the battalion surgeon position	Implement short-term "retraining" before deployment (for subspecialists and nonpracticing MDs) (sick call, trauma, deployed medicine).	Skills and training
	Fill all battalion surgeon PROFIS positions with physician assistants and nurse practitioners (depending on substitutability). (This would require increase in physician assistant/nurse practitioner manning.)	Equity; skills and training; impact on MTFs; retention
	Use a borrowed military manpower system for battalion surgeons. (Providers assigned permanently to battalion surgeon positions, but must work part-time at local MTF.)	Equity; skills and training; impact on MTFs; retention

Table S.1—Continued

Category	Potential Modification	Issues Affected
Improve predictability	Cut orders sooner.	Predictability
	Follow the Army Force Generation (ARFORGEN) cycle for PROFIS positions and personnel. (Do not assign PROFIS personnel to units during reset period of ARFORGEN.)	Equity; predictability; retention
Reduce the impact of deployment on MTFs	Use national backfill contracts to ease hiring challenges at some regional medical commands/MTFs.	Impact on MTFs
Reduce skills degradation	Implement a more formal reassessment of staff skills upon redeployment.	Skills and training; impact on MTFs; retention

Acknowledgments

We gratefully acknowledge the many people in the Office of the Surgeon General, Army Medical Command, the regional medical commands, military treatment facilities and clinics, and elsewhere who graciously took the time to speak with us as part of this project. We also value the contribution of the more than 2,600 men and women in the Army who completed our survey. We appreciate the representatives from allied countries and the U.S. Navy and Air Force who provided us with information about how health care professionals are deployed in their systems.

Thank you also to our Army project officers and points of contact, LTC Shepard Gibson, COL Stephen Sobczak, and COL William Schiek, who provided invaluable assistance throughout the project. We thank Diane Bronowicz for administrative support and the RAND MMIC (Multimode Interviewing Capability) team for support on our survey. We thank Laurie McDonald for preparing the Defense Manpower Data Center data for the project. We thank Dave Baiocchi and Ben Mundell, who graciously provided us with data and expertise from other projects they conducted. Jerry Sollinger provided invaluable help with writing this document. Susan Hosek and Terri Tanielian, co-directors of the Center for Military Health Policy at RAND, provided guidance and support throughout the project—we would not have been successful without their help. We are grateful to the peer reviewers for this document: Ateev Mehrotra, Claude Setodji, and Pete Schirmer. Any errors of fact or interpretation in this report remain the responsibility of the authors.

Abbreviations

ADSO	Active Duty Service Obligation
ALARACT	All Army Activities
AMEDD	Army Medical Department
AOC	area of concentration
ARFORGEN	Army Force Generation
ARTS	Army Medical Department Resource Tasking System
ASI	additional skill identifier
CSH	combat support hospital
DCCS	deputy commander of clinical services
DCN	deputy commander for nursing
ETS	expiration of term of service
FORSCOM	U.S. Army Forces Command
GME	graduate medical education
GSA	Global War on Terrorism Support Assignments
MD	medical doctor
MEDCOM	U.S. Army Medical Command
MOS	military occupation specialty
MTF	military treatment facility
MTOE	Modified Table of Organization and Equipment
OEF	Operation Enduring Freedom
OIF	Operation Iraqi Freedom
OND	Operation New Dawn
PDS	PROFIS Deployment System

PROFIS   Professional Filler System

TDA   Table of Distribution and Allowances

TOE   Table of Organization and Equipment

CHAPTER ONE

Introduction

Background

The Army Medical Department (AMEDD) has multiple missions, including to provide a medical force that supports deployed operations and to deliver health care to soldiers and retirees and their families. The AMEDD does not have enough medical personnel to simultaneously fully staff the requirements it has for both (1) deployable Table of Organization and Equipment (TOE) units, such as combat support hospitals (CSHs) that are under the command of the U.S. Army Forces Command (FORSCOM) and other commands, and (2) Table of Distribution and Allowances (TDA) units, such as military treatment facilities (MTFs), clinics, and other commands on Army bases, which are under the command of the U.S. Army Medical Command (MEDCOM). To accomplish both missions, most medical personnel fill permanent assignments in TDA units, and MEDCOM temporarily reassigns them to fill or augment TOE units with additional medical personnel when these units are preparing for deployment. Upon redeployment, these personnel return to their assigned MTFs (or other assignments). The Professional Filler System (PROFIS) is the regulatory process that MEDCOM uses to identify, assign, train, and qualify professionally trained active Army medical personnel for positions in operating forces (i.e., deploying units).

PROFIS, which covers personnel in the Army Medical, Nurse, Medical Specialist, Dental, Veterinary, Medical Service, and Enlisted Corps, as well as warrant officers, enables health care professionals[1] to work in an MTF performing duties within their specialty when not deployed. This allows the health care professionals to maintain their medical and technical skills. Health care professionals assigned to PROFIS positions are also supposed to maintain their soldier skills, be prepared to deploy when necessary, and periodically train with the TOE units to which they will be assigned when deployed. However, MEDCOM staff report that TDA units do not always release PROFIS personnel for training and that PROFIS personnel frequently reside at different bases from the TOE unit, increasing the challenge of training with the unit. This, in addition to frequent changes in the health care professionals who are assigned to PROFIS slots in TOE units leading up to the time when they deploy, contributes to concerns that PROFIS personnel are not well-trained soldiers, that they are not well integrated with their PROFIS unit when they deploy, and that the system inhibits the deploying unit from developing a meaningful relationship with the health care professionals.

---

[1] We use the term *health care professional* to describe any person with an AMEDD area of concentration (AOC) who is eligible to deploy as a PROFIS filler.

In addition, during the past ten years, the number of deployments for medical personnel has been higher than previously experienced, which has led to some equity issues regarding the frequency and length of deployments. Some specialties, such as surgeons, nurse anesthetists, and physician assistants, deploy at higher rates than other specialties, with many health care professionals in these specialties having deployed multiple times, with standards for dwell time (time at home between deployments) varying with deployment length. Some health care professionals deploy for 12 months, while others deploy for only six months or 90 days.[2] MTF demands and field demands are quite different for many specialties; they require different equipment and consist of different tasks. Some specialized health care professionals worry that their skills degrade while deployed, because of lack of use or a mismatch between the skills needed in the positions they are filling and those that the health care professionals provide.

Although MEDCOM is able to fill all of its PROFIS deployment requirements, AMEDD leaders are concerned that PROFIS is not fully meeting the requirements it was designed to satisfy and that it may have other negative consequences, such as health care professionals becoming dissatisfied with the Army and choosing to leave active duty and potentially reduced access to care at the TDA units when PROFIS health care professionals are deployed.

Purpose and Approach

In light of these concerns, the U.S. Army Surgeon General asked RAND to conduct a study on PROFIS exploring four questions:

- What is the effect of PROFIS on providers?
- What is the effect of PROFIS on nonmedical Army personnel?
- What issues or problems led to the establishment of PROFIS? Do those issues still exist?
- Is an alternative to PROFIS required? What potential improvements are needed?

To answer these four questions, the RAND team developed four tasks. The first was to describe and identify concerns with PROFIS through a literature review and interviews with key stakeholders and AMEDD personnel. The next task was to identify how PROFIS has affected providers by examining existing Army data on deployments and establishing a web-based survey fielded to a sample of AMEDD personnel. The third task was to assess the effect of PROFIS on nonmedical military personnel using the web-based survey, interviews with AMEDD personnel, and coordination with another RAND project measuring the ability of MTFs to meet beneficiary health care during deployments. The fourth task was to identify and assess modifications or alternatives to PROFIS.

We drew on multiple data sources to answer these questions. We interviewed over 100 Army personnel in AMEDD and FORSCOM involved in different aspects of PROFIS, fielded a survey that was completed by over 2,600 health care professionals across seven corps in MEDCOM, analyzed personnel data and PROFIS data on deployments, and collected and

---

[2]   All Army Activities (ALARACT) 253/2007 established a standard dwell time of at least 12 months for combat and operational deployments of 12 months or longer and at least six months for deployments of six months or longer. These dwell times can be waived with a written waiver by a general officer.

analyzed previous reports about PROFIS and MEDCOM deployments. This project was approved by the RAND Institutional Review Board.

How This Report Is Organized

This report describes the results of our research, including describing potential modifications and alternatives to PROFIS. Chapter Two describes PROFIS in more detail, including the regulations that govern PROFIS, how personnel are assigned to PROFIS positions, and a historical timeline of PROFIS. Our data and methods, including the stakeholder interviews, survey, and personnel and deployment data, are discussed in Chapter Three. Drawing on the data and results of the analyses described in Chapter Three, Chapter Four presents the issues and concerns identified from various stakeholders about PROFIS. These include such issues as equity in how the system operates, predictability, skills and training of PROFIS personnel, effect of PROFIS on the MTFs, and retention. Potential modifications or alternatives to the PROFIS that were identified in the literature, interviews, or by the RAND team are described in Chapter Five. Chapter Six presents conclusions and recommendations.[3]

---

[3] This volume also contains three appendixes that provide detail on PROFIS AOCs and how we used them in our analyses. Additional appendixes, which detail results from analyses of corps-specific data, the web survey, and regression analyses, are available at http://www.rand.org/pubs/technical_reports/TR1227.html.

CHAPTER TWO

Background

The Army did not always use PROFIS to manage the deployment of medical personnel. This chapter describes the background and timeline for the development of PROFIS and some of the changes that have occurred to PROFIS over the past decade. We also describe briefly how other services manage deployment of health care professionals, as well as how five of our allies manage these deployments.

The available AMEDD inventory of medical professionals does not allow full staffing of MTFs and TOE units simultaneously. PROFIS was created in 1986 to assign medical officers to MTFs in peacetime and to fill medical positions in deploying units in contingencies (AR 601-142, 1995). This enables medical personnel to maintain their clinical proficiency in the MTFs and to be ready and able to deploy for operations as needed. This resulted in two types of medical positions in modified TOE (MTOE) units: organic positions and PROFIS requirements. Organic positions are required and authorized and are filled by health care professionals that are permanently assigned to the MTOE unit. Examples of typical organic positions include brigade surgeons, leadership positions in the CSHs, and many Army medic positions. Medical positions that are required but not authorized based on the MTOE, or are required and authorized on the MTOE but not supported by the Human Capital Distribution Plan (HCPD), are turned into PROFIS requirements. For some corps (e.g., Army Nurse Corps, Medical Corps) the majority of positions in MTOE units are filled by PROFIS, while for other corps (e.g., Enlisted, Medical Service) the majority are filled by people organic to the unit. PROFIS was initially created as a medical officer filler system for deployable hospitals. Enlisted soldiers were incorporated into PROFIS in 1995, expanding it to include all medical personnel (Leonard, 2002) across 136 AOCs or military occupation specialties (MOSs) in eight corps. Criteria were established for suitable substitutions for specialty requirements (AR 601-142, 1995), which determined the levels of replacement for specialties. Also in 1995, it was determined that a person designated to fill a PROFIS slot would remain in that slot for a minimum of 18 months (AR 601-142, 1995).

Factors Leading to the Development of PROFIS

Following the end of the Korean War, the Army obtained a stable supply of doctors by means of the draft and relied on the Berry Plan to ensure the appropriate mix of specialists. The Berry Plan allowed physicians drafted after completing medical school to delay their service until after completing residency training. Berry Plan participants continued to enter military service for several years after the draft expired. As the Army transitioned to an all-volunteer force in the early 1970s, AMEDD's supply of physicians decreased dramatically. In the 1970s, the Army developed programs, including the physician bonuses, the Health Professions Scholarship Program, a physician's assistants training program, and Uniformed Services University of the Health Sciences (USUHS), to address the decline in providers, yet the Army's supply of physicians reached an all-time low in 1978.[1]

During this time, Major General William P. Winkler, Jr., recommended that AMEDD adopt the Carve/Merge Concept, which formally outlined the procedure for converting the TDA medical requirements into TOEs when necessary. While AMEDD did not ultimately adopt the Carve/Merge Concept, it laid the framework for other policies that would serve this purpose, such as the Korea Medical Augmentation Package (Novier, 1993), which identified Health Services Command as a manpower tool for supporting line units as needed, and the "Staffing Authorization and Utilization of Army Medical Department Commissioned Personnel in Active Component TOE Units of U.S. Army Forces Command (FORSCOM)" letter, commonly known as the MEDO Letter, written by the Office of the Surgeon General. In response to the shortages of medical personnel, the MEDO Letter authorized AMEDD to release the majority of their health care providers from TOE units, allowing them to spend the vast majority of their time working in hospitals and clinics. AMEDD historians consider this to be the beginning of the PROFIS regulations.[2]

In 1983, following the United States' invasion of Grenada (the first contingency operation since the publication of the MEDO Letter), line units that had received clinical fillers from MTFs to support the mission issued complaints about the timeliness of receiving medical personnel into the unit and the medical personnel's low readiness and lack of familiarity with unit operations and procedures, due to their absence during the unit's training (Nolan, 1990). This was the impetus for implementing Army Regulation (AR) 601-142, *Army Medical Department Professional Officer Filler System*, in 1986, which officially established PROFIS and described PROFIS as a system with responsibility shared between the Army Surgeon General and the Army Military Personnel Center commander.

PROFIS Overview

AR 601-142 governs the PROFIS program. It outlines specific responsibilities for key individuals involved in managing the program and provides guidance on matters such as training. In accordance with the regulation, both the providing and gaining units share the responsibility to ensure that PROFIS personnel are trained and ready to perform their critical wartime skills. The first publication of AR 601-142 was August 15, 1986, establishing the policies and procedures for the PROFIS program. The regulation established guidelines for the active component officers who were mobilized through PROFIS to fill positions in FORSCOM for early deployed or forward deployed forces in Europe and Korea (AR 601-142, 1986). In this original regulation, PROFIS personnel were required to report to their deploying unit within 72 hours of notification, and positions could be filled by officers whose ranks were two above or two below what the TOE called for (AR 601-142, 1986). Currently, PROFIS personnel join their

---

[1]   Correspondence with Army historians.

[2]   Correspondence with Army historians.

deploying units no more than 30 days prior to the expected date of deployment, and positions can be filled by officers whose ranks are two above or one below the position (AR 601-142, 2007).

MEDCOM developed the PROFIS Deployment System (PDS) in 2005 to improve the predictability and equity of PROFIS deployments in the current rotational deployment environment. PDS is a selection and management system within PROFIS that is used to fill requirements with the appropriate personnel for units scheduled to deploy usually within the following year. PDS allows for the more central management of PROFIS requirements for upcoming deployments. PDS separates health care professionals by AOC (officers) or MOS (enlisted personnel) into three tiers based on their numbers and deployment schedule (see Appendix A for the AOCs/MOSs in each tier); additional skill identifiers (ASIs) are also used in the placement of some AOCs. The tier determines the process used to fill taskings for AOCs/MOSs. Tier I includes 39 low-density AOCs/MOSs that have a large impact on AMEDD missions (e.g., general surgeon, physician assistant, social worker). Tier I slots are managed centrally by MEDCOM. Tier II includes 46 AOCs/MOSs (e.g., pediatrician, general dentist, physical therapist) whose PROFIS deployments are managed at the AMEDD major subordinate command level, primarily by the regional (medical, dental, etc.) commands.[3] Tier III consists of 49 AOCs/MOSs that are more prevalent or less frequently deployed (e.g., preventive medicine officer, health care administrator, field veterinary service officer, health care specialist [combat medic]). Selecting Tier III personnel for deployment is performed by the MTF,[4] though the regional medical command can decide to take on this role.

MEDCOM works closely with AOC consultants, who are subject-matter experts for their AOC and are appointed by the Army Surgeon General, in the selection of personnel to fill the Tier I requirements. MEDCOM determines the distribution of Tier II and Tier III requirements among the regional medical commands, taking into consideration primarily each regional medical command's assigned strength within each AOC. MEDCOM also performs the daily management of PROFIS and PDS, including managing replacements and reclamas; holds the annual PDS conference at which Tier I positions are filled; and develops PROFIS policy (U.S. Army Medical Command, 2011).

The developers of PROFIS did not anticipate the current conflicts involving rotational deployment of units. An ongoing schedule has been developed for managing PROFIS assignments for Operation Enduring Freedom (OEF)/Operation Iraqi Freedom (OIF)/Operation New Dawn (OND) and other contingency rotations. Approximately eight months before the first unit in a new rotational schedule will deploy, MEDCOM verifies the requirements for PROFIS personnel in all the units that will deploy, including medical augmentees that have been identified, and these requirements are moved into PDS. Individual augmentees that support enduring missions are identified during the same timeframe. Augmentees are those positions that have been identified as being required for a mission but that are not on the original TOE for the unit deploying. Approximately six months before the start of the new rotation when a group of units will deploy, an annual PDS conference is held at which individual per-

---

[3]   There are currently five regional medical commands: three are in the continental United States (Northern, Southern, and Western Regional Medical Commands) in addition to Pacific and Europe Regional Medical Commands. In the remainder of this report, when we refer to regional medical commands, we are also referring to other major subordinate commands that provide PROFIS personnel, such as Public Health Command and Medical Research and Materiel Command.

[4]   There are 39 MTFs located across the five regional medical commands.

sonnel are assigned to fill the required Tier I positions. Tier II/III requirements are distributed to the regional medical commands, which in turn distribute Tier III requirements to individual MTFs and clinics for the selection of personnel to fill each required position. Approximately five months before the start of a new rotation, the list of health care professionals filling PDS requirements is "locked." Subsequent changes to the person identified to fill a requirement involve a reclama, which is a formal declination request from a clinic, MTF, or regional medical command that requires MEDCOM approval. Reclamas can occur for a variety of reasons, such as the identification of a profile (e.g., injury, medical condition) rendering the person temporarily or permanently nondeployable, the critical position the person has at the MTF, or the inability to backfill a position where the number of other providers of the same AOC is very limited at the MTF from which the provider is being deployed. MEDCOM conducts an electronic-based PDS conference approximately six months after the in-person PDS conference to assign people to PROFIS slots that have been identified since the in-person PDS conference as deploying soon.

Typically, the consultants or the permanent duty station that health care professionals are based at notify them that they have been selected for a PROFIS deployment. They also receive an email in their Army Knowledge Online account when their name has been locked into a position. MEDCOM policy requires this notification to occur within 15 days of the health care professional being selected to fill a requirement and at least 30 days prior to actual deployment (U.S. Army Medical Command, 2011). If notified less than 30 days before scheduled to deploy, the health care professional has the option of joining the unit 30 days later in their deployed location. PROFIS health care professionals are officially attached to the deploying unit by a Temporary Change of Station order.

The percentage of deployments of health care professionals during contingencies that are filled by PROFIS personnel compared with organic personnel varies substantially across the corps (Figure 2.1). PROFIS deployments range from less than 10 percent of deployments in the Enlisted Corps to more than 75 percent of deployments in the Nurse Corps during OEF/OIF.[5] The portion of PROFIS deployments in each corps depends on the percentage of the corps deployed through PROFIS and on the relative size of the corps. For example, although a small portion of the enlisted deployments are filled by PROFIS, deployments from the very large Enlisted Corps make up 32 percent of all PROFIS deployments (Figure 2.2), which is slightly more than either the Medical or Nurse Corps.[6]

Turmoil in the System

Over the course of OEF/OIF, the composition of PROFIS personnel who actually deploy has shifted from the requirements listed for units in the MTOE as unit commanders have made the determination that operational needs require a different mix of skills. Commanders have therefore dropped PROFIS positions for some AOCs and added positions for other AOCs— for example, adding a pediatrician to a CSH if part of its mission is treating Afghani villagers.

---

[5]   These are approximations as the number of PROFIS deployments and the number of total deployments was derived from different data sources (Army Medical Department Resource Tasking System [ARTS] and Defense Manpower Data Center [DMDC] data, respectively).

[6]   Based on ARTS data and limited to deployments that were more than one month in duration.

Figure 2.1
Percentage of All Deployments of Health Care Professionals During OEF/OIF (2002–2009) Filled by
PROFIS Personnel, by Corps

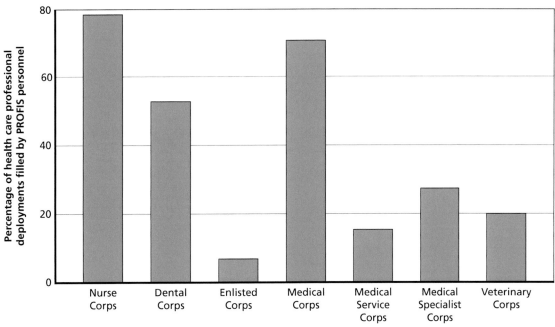

RAND *TR1227-2.1*

Figure 2.2
Distribution of PROFIS Deployments During OEF/OIF Across Corps
(2002–2009)

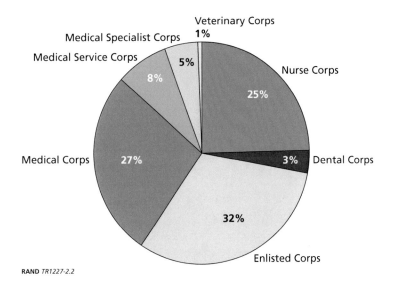

RAND *TR1227-2.2*

These added positions that do not appear on the TOE are considered *medical augmentees* (not required on the MTOE, but considered essential for the mission) or *individual augmentees* (validated by Army Headquarters operations and plans for special or unique missions), but are still managed through PROFIS and PDS.[7] Currently, instead of using the TOE, MEDCOM uses the currently deployed force in the planning of PROFIS requirements for the next unit deploying. However, commanders for upcoming deployments may subsequently decide to deploy with fewer of the PROFIS personnel assigned to their unit, at which point these PROFIS personnel can be released and might be available for reassignment to other PROFIS requirements. This may occur after personnel have been notified by their AOC consultant or MTF leadership that they have been selected for deployment. Alternatively, a unit commander can request to augment the unit with additional PROFIS personnel if there is additional need for the skills of a specific specialty. These individuals are also handled as individual augmentees; the identification of the additional requirements and assignment of personnel may occur substantially after the PDS conference. Ideally, commanders are supposed to make an official request for their PROFIS fillers, including all augmentees, at least 60 days prior to deployment (AR 601-142, 2007).

Changes to Deployment Length for PROFIS Personnel During OEF/OIF

The length of time that PROFIS fillers have deployed has varied over time and by corps. Here we highlight ALARACT messages that affect PROFIS assignments and deployment length. Figure 2.3 shows events that affect demand for medical personnel on the bottom and the dates of policies affecting health care professional deployments on the top. Starting in 1995, the policy stated that individuals would be assigned to PROFIS positions for 18 months (AR 601-142, 1995)—this was not related to deployment length, rather it referred to how long they should be assigned to a position.[8] Until 2004, PROFIS personnel would deploy for the entire time their unit was deploying, which could vary depending on the mission, but was often 12 months, especially during OEF. Concerns about skills degradation for both specialists and primary care physicians during often year-long deployments were prevalent for a number of reasons. MTF demands and field demands are quite different; they require different equipment and consist of different tasks. During deployment, providers do not have the opportunity to practice medicine as they would in an MTF or their stateside care setting (Sarmiento, 2004). Many physicians also felt underutilized on deployments, particularly if they were serving outside of their trained specialty, and expressed concern that this would degrade their clinical skills (Edgar, 2009).

In June 2004, the 180-Day AMEDD PROFIS/Individual Augmentee (IA) Rotation Policy was published (ALARACT 108/2004). This allowed two health care professionals to split a deployment, with each person deploying for approximately 180 days. It applied only to a subset of specialized AOCs in the Medical, Dental, and Nurse Corps[9] serving in PROFIS

---

[7] For the purpose of this report, we use the term *PROFIS deployment* for any deployment managed through PROFIS, including medical augmentees, individual augmentees, and active- to reserve-component deployments.

[8] The 2007 update to AR 601-142 did not contain an analogous policy on the length of assignment to PROFIS positions.

[9] 61K, 61Z, 60B, 60F, 60G, 60H (interventionists), 60J, 60K, 60L, 60M, 60N, 60P (subspecialists), 60Q, 60R, 60S, 60T, 60V, 61A, 61B, 61C, 61D, 61G, 61J, 61L, 61M, 61P, 61R, 61U, 61W, 63D, 63E, 63F, 63N, and 66F.

Figure 2.3
Changes to PROFIS/PDS During OEF/OIF

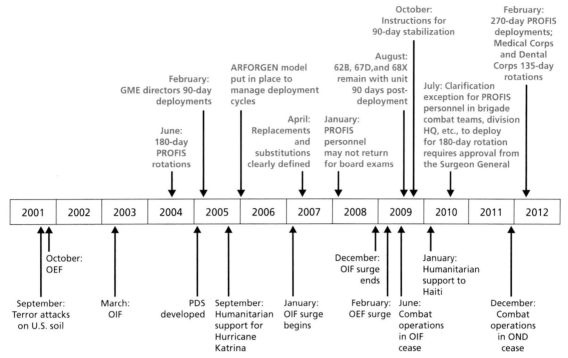

NOTE: GME = graduate medical education.
RAND TR1227-2.3

assignments in echelon-above-division units, level 3 MTFs, or forward surgical teams and required a minimum of 30 days of notification for individual replacements with the goal of having replacements arrive around 180 days into the deployment.[10] Other health care professionals (both organic and PROFIS) remained for the entire deployment, typically 12 to 15 months. In February 2005, an addendum was published to the 180-Day Rotation Policy that increased its flexibility and made more individuals eligible to request exemptions for 180-day deployments. It also added that graduate medical education (GME) directors could deploy for 90 days and specified that the approving authority for exception to policy requests regarding length of deployments was through the deployed chain of command to the theater surgeon, MEDCOM, and then approved by the assistant surgeon general for force projection.

In January 2008, ALARACT 005/2008, entitled "180-Day Professional Filler System Deployment Policy ISO OIF/OEF," was published, with the goal to help mitigate the degradation of complex medical, dental, and nursing skills not practiced in combat zones; the policy expanded eligibility for 180-day deployments to all AOCs in the Medical, Dental, and Nurse Corps serving in units echelon-above-brigade, level 3 MTFs, or forward surgical teams. It also directed that anyone who was deployed as a 180-day rotator could not return from deployment early in order to take specialty board certification examinations. This had the potential to

---

[10] For AOCs eligible for 180-day deployments, both the initial deployer and the replacement are typically identified at the PDS conference for Tier I requirements.

affect the pool of possible deployers, as the consultants and commanders would avoid scheduling for deployment individuals planning to take board exams.

In March 2009, MEDCOM released a policy memorandum addressing PROFIS/individual augmentee replacements (Schoomaker, 2009). This policy allowed for specified individuals to request replacements once in theater through their chain of command if there were more than 90 days remaining on the unit's deployment, in order to return to begin graduate medical education, long-term health education and training programs, and AOC/MOS-producing schools longer than 180 days. It also enabled GME directors to return after 90 days. In addition, the policy allowed those who were not 180-day rotators to request replacements in order to return for board/licensure examinations. The policy was further formalized in March 2011, when it was replaced by MEDCOM 11-024 (Schoomaker, 2011).

Increasing awareness of and concerns about the impact of deployment on the mental health of soldiers led to ALARACT 214/2009. To sustain their support for redeploying soldiers, field surgeons (62B),[11] behavioral sciences officers (67D), and behavioral health specialists (68X) attached to brigade combat teams deploying on or after August 1, 2009, were to remain with their deploying unit for a minimum of 90 days upon return from deployment. Because the majority of PROFIS fillers do not come from the same base as the deploying unit, this policy caused those three specialties to be away from their home station well beyond their deployment time, for a total of 9 to 15 months, depending on the duration of their unit's deployment and whether their rotation had been split. An addendum was published in October 2009 that allowed for exception to policies to include the additional 90 days in determining the duration of split rotations (15-month deployments could be split at the 7.5-month point) for those designated personnel assigned to brigade combat teams (ALARACT 214/2009 and Addendum to ALARACT 214/2009).

To align with the Army's 270-day deployment length policy, ALARACT 013/2012 established a 270-day deployment period for PROFIS deployments starting in February 2012. Medical Corps and Dental Corps officers now deploy for 135 days if assigned to PROFIS positions in medical brigades or units echelon above brigade. Exceptions include Medical Corps officers serving in a deputy commander for clinical services or a deputy commander for administration position and Medical Corps or Dental Corps officers assigned or attached to a division headquarters who will deploy for 270 days.

Deployment of Medical Personnel in Other Services

Each of the services uses slightly different procedures and policies for managing medical forces deployments. Here, we briefly describe the U.S. Navy and U.S. Air Force systems.

Navy

The Navy Bureau of Medicine and Surgery uses three programs to fill deployment taskings: Health Services Augmentation Program, Individual Augmentation Manpower Management, and Global War on Terrorism Support Assignments, which were replaced by Overseas Contingency Operation Support Assignments in October 2010. The requests for the Health Services Augmentation Program and Individual Augmentation Manpower Management sourcing are

---

[11] The majority of field surgeon deployments are as battalion surgeons.

sent out to the four Navy medical regional commands. Each region has been tasked to support specific missions as a region as well as health care operations in their geographic area, which is similar to how the AMEDD manages Tier II PROFIS requirements. Like Tier I PROFIS requirements, taskings for low-density, high-demand occupations may be filled across regions (BUMEDISNT, 2007).

The Health Services Augmentation Program is an active-duty-only program that allows the Navy to pull medical personnel from MTFs in order to provide intra-service support to the Marine Corps and also support Navy operations. Under the Health Services Augmentation Program, if a regional command is unable to fill all of its assigned taskings, it is required to provide a by-name list of all qualified personnel within the command along with a justification for why they cannot deploy within ten days of receipt of the tasking (Department of Navy, 2010). Then a reclama process is used to fill these slots from a different region.

Individual Augmentation Manpower Management identifies individual augmentees to fill joint requirements in the U.S. Central Command area of responsibility from either the active or reserve components. Global War on Terrorism Support Assignments are active duty–only positions and are managed by Navy Military Personnel Command. These assignments are only available to medical personnel who are negotiating their permanent change of station orders.

A very small number of non-residency-trained physicians (general medical officers) are used in the deployed setting for the Navy, and they are managed under the Individual Augmentation or Health Services Augmentation programs. Most Navy general medical officers fill organic billets on Navy ships or in Marine Corps battalions. The general medical officers are targeted for these jobs. Typically, there are two organic physician slots in these units, and one will be filled with a general medical officer and the other with a specialty physician.

Naval Medical Command Policy 09-010 states that sailors should receive a minimum of 60-day notice, though operational needs may require a shorter notification time. Typically the notification to medical personnel occurs 80–120 days prior to deployment (Robinson, 2009).

Deployments for Navy personnel are typically 210 days for Health Services Augmentation Program and Individual Augmentation deployments in addition to predeployment training. The Global War on Terrorism Support/Operational Support Assignment deployments vary in length between six and 14 months and are tied to a permanent change of station move. Medical specialists, such as general surgeons, anesthesiologists, and nurse anesthetists, may have shorter deployments. Unlike many PROFIS deployments, the Navy typically requires its personnel to deploy for the entire amount of time and does not allow medical personnel to return from the U.S. Central Command area of responsibility to take board exams. However, for hospital ship missions or theater security cooperation missions, the Navy will send more than one person to fill a requirement, essentially shortening deployments for these individuals. Standards for dwell time are a minimum of six months (BUMEDINST, 2007).

Air Force

Unlike the Army, the Air Force Medical Service (AFMS) uses a modular structure called the Expeditionary Medical Support (EMEDS) system for deployments. The EMEDS system can be used to deploy health care professionals in structures from small teams, such as the Squadron Medical Element (three health care professionals) and Global Reach Laydown team (four health care professionals) to an Air Force theater hospital with 25 inpatient beds (Medical Annex to AFI 10-401, 2010). Requirements are identified for specific capabilities, which are then associated with standard deployable unit type codes (UTCs). Larger expeditionary medical units, such as an Air Force theater hospital, are composed of combinations of UTCs.

While unit commanders who are health care professionals are organic to the expeditionary medical units, other health care professionals who are assigned to UTCs are permanently assigned to Air Force MTFs in order to provide them with a clinical caseload to maintain skills (Medical Annex to AFI 10-401, 2010). Health care professionals assigned to a particular UTC are typically all assigned to the MTF, when not deployed, which facilitates the building of teamwork within a UTC. However, not all of the UTCs required for a larger expeditionary medical unit are co-located with a single MTF. Furthermore, individuals within a UTC may be deployed to different locations, or only some health care professionals assigned to a UTC may be deployed if required by the mission.

Deployments for Air Force health care professionals are typically 180 days; leadership positions may be 365 days. Most of the Air Force medical personnel have a 1:3 deployment-to-dwell-time ratio, deploying six months every 24 months. However, mental health providers have a 1:2 deployment-to-dwell ratio, deploying six months every 18 months. The Air Force may use physicians who have not completed residency training as flight surgeons when critically short of physicians to fill authorizations.

All personnel have a six-month deployment vulnerability period during which they may be deployed, even if they are not assigned to a UTC (AFI 10-401, 2010). Within their vulnerability period, Air Force personnel are instructed to be prepared to deploy at any time. With this system, the Air Force attempts to eliminate any short-notice deployments for personnel during their vulnerability period. Unit deployment managers assign available personnel to authorized positions in UTCs up to 24 months out. Air Force personnel are typically aware at least six months ahead that they will deploy. Health care professionals who are not assigned to a UTC, but are within their vulnerability period, may fill in for those who cannot deploy for some reason, such as not being medically ready.

The Air Force tries to balance deployment requirements and skills in selected occupations primarily the low-supply, high-demand specialties, using the Consultant Balanced Deployment program. Medical specialists included in the program include emergency physicians and nurses, critical care physicians and nurses, surgeons, mental health providers, nurse anesthetists, and operating room nurses (Medical Annex to AFI 10-401, 2010).

Predeployment training varies by UTC. All health care professionals are supposed to be fully qualified in the skills required for their UTC prior to entering their vulnerability period for deployment. Requirements for predeployment training are specified in their deployment instructions (orders) and vary by UTC and deployment (AFI 41-106, 2011).

Deployment of Medical Personnel in Selected Other Countries

Other countries take different approaches to deploying medical personnel. To inform potential modifications to PROFIS, we sought information on some of these approaches. Here, we briefly summarize the approaches taken by five countries: Canada, Germany, the Netherlands, Sweden, and the United Kingdom. This information was compiled through interviews, written communication, and literature review.

Differences in Health Care Systems

There are important differences in the health care systems of these countries that may limit the comparability and applicability of medical personnel management to the U.S. system. Where possible, these differences have been identified (see Table 2.1). One of the most important differences is that these five countries have some form of national health care system, while the United States does not (OECD, 2010). This difference may influence the dynamics between the military and civilian health care sectors.

How Services Are Provided to Armed Forces

The Canadian Forces Health Services Group includes approximately 6,400 regular force, reserve force, and civilian personnel and 500 civilian contractors. The Canadian Forces Health Services Group is designed as a joint support unit that serves all service branches (i.e., Army, Air Force, and Navy). Health Services personnel are designated to a particular service but may work in different service branches. For example, a Canadian Forces Medical Services nurse could be designated to the Army yet still be assigned to deploy with the Air Force. In Canada, military personnel receive primary medical care and dental care at military base clinics, health care centers, and support units. More complex medical care (e.g., specialist care, hospital care, after-hours medical care) is generally provided in civilian health care facilities. Most military physicians work almost exclusively in civilian hospitals when not deployed, but may have clinic at a military base once a week. Military medical training is also largely provided in the civilian setting.

Medical personnel for the German armed forces, the *Bundeswehr*, are assigned to a centralized authority of the Joint Medical Service, which is responsible for military hospitals, health care centers, and consultant centers. Military personnel receive care primarily from military providers in military installations. Civilian physicians may contract with the government to provide medical care to military personnel as well. Dependents and civil employees of the armed forces utilize the civilian medical system.

The Royal Netherlands Forces Health Care Organizations currently include approximately 3,600 regular personnel (2,800 military and 800 civilian) and 300 reservists, though this number is to be reduced by almost 25 percent. They provide medical services to regular and reserve forces military personnel. While primary care and general medicine military physicians work in military health care centers while not deployed, specialists work in civilian medical care settings to maintain their clinical skills. Military hospital care, rehabilitative center care, dental care, physiotherapy, part of pharmacy, and part of curative care are insured within the military health care system. Care for military personnel received from civilian health care institutions is also paid through this military medical insurance system. Military dependents use the civilian medical system.

The Swedish Armed Forces Health Service include approximately 1,300 regular force, reserve force, and civilian personnel. These people provide health care and medical services to regular and reserve forces personnel. However, most military medical personnel work in civilian hospitals.

The Defence Medical Group (DMG), which is responsible for overseeing all British Army, Royal Air Force, and Royal Navy medical staff, oversees approximately 1,800 regular medical staff. The individual services are each responsible for delivering primary health care to military personnel and medical support for operations. Most military providers work in the National Health Service (NHS) and are considered regular NHS staff, although their salary is paid in

Table 2.1
Comparison of Health Care Systems, Physician Employment, Mandatory Military Service, and Provision of Medical Care to Military Populations for Selected Allied Countries

Country	National Health Care System	Are Physicians Employed by Government or Private Sector?*	Mandatory Military Service (Conscription)[a]	Sector That Provides Primary Care to Military	Sector That Provides Secondary/ Specialist/ Hospital Care to Military	Are Civilian Health Care Professionals Deployed?	Average Length of Deployment
United States	No	Private	No	Military	Primarily Military	No	6 months to 1 year; 90 days for GME directors
Canada	Yes	Predominantly private	No	Hybrid	Hybrid	Yes, volunteers	6 months; 6–8 weeks for surgeons
Germany	Yes	Hybrid, largely private	Yes**	Hybrid	Hybrid	No	4 months
The Netherlands	Yes	Private	No	Hybrid	Hybrid	Yes, specialists	4 to 6 months; 6 weeks to 4 months for surgical teams and specialists
Sweden	Yes	Private with government contracts	No	Civilian	Civilian	No	6 months; 6 to 8 weeks for surgical teams
United Kingdom	Yes	Hybrid, largely government	No	Hybrid	Hybrid	No	6 months, including predeployment training

* OECD, 2010.

** Germany ended conscription on July 1, 2011.

[a] ChartsBin, 2010; War Resisters, 2009; Central Intelligence Agency, 2010.

part by the Ministry of Defence. When a military hospital deploys, clinical staff are drawn from across all three armed services to deploy to the field hospitals. Clinicians are selected for deployment first from local Territorial Army resources and subsequently from national Territorial Army and regular medical staff from the armed forces.

Personnel Deployed

Several of the countries interviewed reported deploying civilian medical personnel. For example, due to a reported shortage of some types of specialists in the military, the Canadian Forces Health System has been deploying civilian volunteers since 2006 for specialties where shortages exist. The Canadian Forces use financial incentives to promote civilian physician deployments; however, based on our interviewee's opinion, many of the civilian medical providers are unprepared for military medical care because they do not understand the intricacies of providing medical care in a combat setting.

The Netherlands also deploys civilian medical personnel through a unique reciprocity arrangement through which the Defence Agency has approximately 80 military medical specialists working in civilian hospitals and in return approximately 180 civilian medical specialists deploy for short time periods. The civilian personnel have basic military training and the status of a reservist. This arrangement allows the military medical specialists to maintain their clinical and surgical skills while also providing a larger number of personnel for deployment. Assignments for the more challenging deployments are restricted only to military medical personnel.

In Sweden, most military medical personnel work in civilian hospitals. They spend most of their time as civilians and become military personnel only during deployment. Medical personnel formally volunteer to deploy through the Armed Forces website.

Length of Deployment

Most country contacts reported that medical personnel deploy for six months or less, although the length of deployment varies by country and by type of medical personnel. In Canada, medical technicians, general duty (family medicine) physicians, nurses, and physician assistants typically have six-month deployments. Specialist physicians may deploy for the full six months; however, most surgeons deploy for only six to eight weeks. Civilian deployments average four weeks.

The average reported duration of deployment for German medical personnel was four months. Medical personnel in specialties with a high demand split deployments, resulting in deployment lengths of two months or even less, but personnel in Ready Battalions, Quick Reaction Forces, and at headquarters serve six-month tours that are not split.

The average reported deployment period in the Netherlands was between four to six months, depending on the mission and type of medical personnel. Surgical teams and medical care specialists have shorter rotation periods, ranging from six weeks up to four months. The civilian medical specialists have the shortest deployments, ranging from six weeks to three months.

In Sweden, deployments typically last six months. However, surgical teams (surgeon, anesthesiologist, scrub nurse, and anesthetic nurse) normally deploy for only six to eight weeks. In the United Kingdom, medical personnel deploy for six months but receive operation-specific training prior to deployment, which is included in the total deployment length.

CHAPTER THREE

Data and Methods

This report uses four distinct types of data: interviews with Army personnel in AMEDD and FORSCOM involved in different aspects of PROFIS; data from a survey of health care professionals across seven corps in MEDCOM; Army Medical Department Resource Tasking System (ARTS) data on PROFIS deployments; and Defense Manpower Data Center administrative data that track Army personnel. This chapter describes the data, how we collected them, and the approaches we took to analyze the information.

Key-Informant Interviews

We conducted semistructured key-informant interviews[1] as part of the project task focused on identifying concerns with the performance of PROFIS in the current operating environment. The research team conducted interviews with a purposefully selected group of stakeholders, including those involved in the management and operation of PROFIS at MEDCOM, at the regional medical commands, and at individual MTFs; consultants to the Army Surgeon General; MTF commanders; clinical leadership (e.g., deputy commander of clinical services (DCCS), deputy commander for nursing (DCN)) and clinical staff stationed at Army medical centers and clinics, including Walter Reed Army Medical Center, Carl R. Darnall Army Medical Center, Brook Army Medical Center, Womack Army Medical Center, Madigan Army Medical Center, and Guthrie Ambulatory Clinic; GME program directors; Office of the Surgeon General staff; and staff at Medical Research and Materiel Command, U.S. Army Dental Command, and U.S. Army Veterinary Command, as well as at four of the regional medical commands: Western Regional Medical Command, Northern Regional Medical Command, Southern Regional Medical Command, and Pacific Regional Medical Command.

In addition to gaining information on how PROFIS functions, we sought to obtain insight into how PROFIS affects health care professionals and MTFs. Interview topics included those listed below:

- communication with AOC consultants
- how health care professionals are selected for deployments
- issues with individual augmentees
- alignment between health care professional skills and deployed clinical activities

---

[1] Semistructured interviews use a set of themes or open-ended questions as a starting point, but allow the interviewer to bring up new questions or modify or eliminate planned questions as a result of interviewee responses.

- recruiting and retention of health care professionals
- duration and frequency of deployments
- notification of upcoming deployments
- training for deployments
- reintegration of health care professionals upon return to the MTF
- skills degradation
- impact of deployments on the MTF
- suggestions for improving PROFIS.

We also conducted semistructured key-informant interviews with personnel assigned to FORSCOM units, including senior commanders, CSH commanders, division surgeons, brigade combat team commanders and command sergeant majors, and brigade and battalion surgeons at Fort Hood, Fort Lewis, Fort Sam Houston, Fort Bragg, Fort Shafter, and Fort Campbell, to gain their perspective and insights into PROFIS. Following a similar protocol, we probed issues about individual augmentees, selecting PROFIS personnel, notification and training, how well PROFIS personnel integrated into the unit and how well their skills matched the demands of the deployment, split deployments, the importance of the 90-day post-deployment stabilization period, and thoughts on the way PROFIS could be improved.

The majority of interviews were conducted in person, with a few occurring by videoconference or telephone. Each interview involved two members of the research team, with one team member conducting the interview and the other taking notes, which were then reviewed by the interviewer for completeness. Three team members, including both project leaders, developed a coding classification system. A single team member coded and analyzed the interview notes using Atlas.ti version 6.2 to ensure consistency in coding. To ensure completeness and accuracy of coding, after the first ten interviews were coded, both project leaders reviewed the coding and discussed and resolved any discrepancies in coding. The project leads resolved questions about coding on an ongoing basis.

We interviewed 117 individuals. Of these, 36 represented FORSCOM personnel (22 medical and 14 nonmedical), 13 represented the regional medical commands, 46 represented MTFs, and 16 represented the Office of the Surgeon General or MEDCOM. Among these, eight were consultants to the Army Surgeon General for PROFIS. We also spoke with three individuals with Dental Corps and three individuals with Veterinary Corps. In addition, we conducted briefings for a variety of audiences throughout the project and received feedback and more information during these briefings. The briefing audiences included the command sergeant majors in MEDCOM, MEDCOM general officers and/or their staff, and attendees at the 2011 PDS conference.

The results from the interviews, which are discussed throughout Chapter Four, informed the design of our analytic strategies for the remainder of the project. Table 3.1 shows the key issues identified through the interviews and indicates the other data sources used to assess these issues.

Survey

We conducted a web-based survey of a stratified random sample of health care professionals to assess views and experiences with PROFIS. A preliminary literature review and the interviews

Table 3.1
Key Issues Identified During Interviews and Data Used to Assess

Category	Issues Identified in Interviews	Survey	ARTS Data	Personnel Data
Equity	Who is deploying			X
	Number of times individuals deploy			X
	Length of deployment	X	X	X
	Type of deployments	X	X	
	Battalion surgeon positions	X	X	
Predictability	Short notice for deployment	X		
	Health care professional assigned to PROFIS position keeps changing			
Skills and training	Skills mismatch	X	X	
	Underutilization/low caseload in specialty	X		
Impact on MTFs	Increased workload	X		
	Perception of reduced access	X		
Retention	Impact of deployments on retention and intention to remain in military	X		X

described above with current PROFIS personnel, health care professionals, and other Army leaders informed the survey development. Recently retired Army medical personnel reviewed the survey wording and response options to ensure the question wording, response options, and survey length were appropriate for the target population. We selected retired individuals because we could utilize their familiarity with the topics being addressed and population of interest, without decreasing the size of our potential sample. The RAND Institutional Review Board (IRB) and a Department of Defense Second Level Review approved the survey.

Survey Items

The survey focused on three broad topics: (1) the impact of PROFIS on health care professionals, (2) current issues/problems with PROFIS and PDS, and (3) potential improvements to PROFIS. The survey asked specific questions to address the main research questions. Table 3.2 includes examples of questions included in the survey. The survey used five-point scales (e.g., very satisfied, satisfied, neither satisfied nor dissatisfied, dissatisfied, very dissatisfied; very important, important, neither important nor unimportant, unimportant, very unimportant) to measure perceptions. Survey questions included "Don't know" and "Not applicable" responses where appropriate.

The survey also included basic background questions to understand PROFIS from a variety of AMEDD personnel perspectives. Background information collected included rank, MOS or AOC, ASIs, amount of time spent in the Army as an active duty soldier, prior military experience, method of entrance into the Army (Health Professions Scholarship Program, Reserve Officers' Training Corps, United States Military Academy, etc.), permanent duty station, number of deployments, and most recent deployment experience (length of deployment, type of unit during deployment, PROFIS status, month and year of most recent deployment,

Table 3.2
Categories of Questions from PROFIS Survey

The Impact of PROFIS on AMEDD Personnel
How satisfied are PROFIS personnel with their integration into the unit they deployed with?
How satisfied are individuals with the integration and proficiency of PROFIS personnel assigned to their unit?
How satisfied are PROFIS personnel with the initial notification of deployment and the time between receipt of official orders and deployment?
How important are different types of trainings for PROFIS providers?
How do the number and/or length of deployments affect medical personnel's clinical/surgical/procedural and/or leadership skills?
Current Issues/Problems with PROFIS and PDS
What are the respondents' general perceptions of PROFIS including equity of the system and their relationship with their consultant?
What is the impact of PROFIS of the MTF and/or home station clinic?
What is the impact of PROFIS on retention of Army medical personnel?
Potential Improvements to PROFIS
How can PROFIS be improved?

number of years out of residency at time of deployment, and board certification status at time of deployment).

Survey Eligibility and Sampling

The survey population included individuals in the active duty Army in November 2010 and with an AOC/MOS that identified them as being in any of the following AMEDD corps: Enlisted Corps, Medical Corps, Dental Corps, Veterinary Corps, Medical Specialist Corps, Nurse Corps, and Medical Service Corps. Personnel identified as interns (9E ASI) or residents (9D ASI) who were in training units were excluded from the population. Thirty individuals without an Army email address were excluded. The Enlisted, Dental, Veterinary, Specialist, and Nurse Corps each formed a stratum. Multiple strata were created within the Medical Service Corps (two strata) and Medical Corps (eight strata) to ensure adequate representation of certain AOCs. The grouping of AOCs into strata is presented in Appendix B. Within each stratum, a simple random sample without replacement was drawn; the sampling probability varied by stratum (Table 3.3). A minimum sample of 200 individuals was selected for each corps. Within the Medical Corps, the sampling probability was increased from 50 percent to 70 percent for strata that were to be included in subanalyses if 50 percent yielded a sample of fewer than 300 individuals.

Survey Dissemination

An invitation to participate was emailed to the AMEDD medical personnel in the survey sample by the RAND Corporation's MultiMode Interview Capability (MMIC). Weekly email reminders were sent to individuals who had not yet responded to participate in the survey for the first three weeks following the initial invitation, with a reminder letter mailed a month after the initiation of the survey. The survey was available online from December 1, 2010, until

Table 3.3
Survey Sample Size, by Strata

Corps	Population Size	Number in Sample	Percentage of Population Included in Sample
Enlisted Corps	36,119	2,000	6
Medical Corps	4,293	2,436	56
Family medicine and substitutes	1,509	751	50
Subspecialty, procedure-intensive	400	277	70
Subspecialty, non-procedure-intensive	742	368	50
Nondirect patient care	365	180	50
General surgery	298	208	70
General surgery substitutes	368	254	70
Specialty surgery	468	326	70
Other	143	72	50
Dental Corps	951	300	32
Veterinary Corps	491	200	41
Medical Specialist Corps	1,501	500	33
Nurse Corps	3,960	1,500	38
Medical Service Corps	4,790	1,000	21
Behavioral health specialists	388	272	70
Other specialists	4,402	728	17

February 1, 2011. The average survey completion time was approximately 15 minutes. A total of 2,610 individuals completed the survey. The overall response rate was 33 percent, ranging from 14 percent in the Enlisted Corps to 51 percent in the Veterinary Corps (Table 3.4).

Survey Analyses

We developed a conceptual model to guide our analysis of the survey data (Figure 3.1). The three main outcomes of interest were perceptions of PROFIS, impact of PROFIS on the MTFs, and intentions to remain in the military. We hypothesized that these outcomes would be affected by health care professionals' "deployment experience," which encompasses the full spectrum of preparing for deployment (e.g., training performed prior to deployment, timing of notification for deployment); characteristics of the deployment (e.g., number of times deployed, deployed as a 62B or as another AOC, length of deployment, extent to which provider felt clinically prepared for deployment); the redeployment experience[2] (e.g., how long the individual remained with deploying unit upon return to the United States, views

---

[2]   Due to a lack of variation in the redeployment experience variables, we were unable to include these variables in the regression models. We do, however, include redeployment bivariate results in Appendix K.

Table 3.4
Response Rate, by Corps (as compared with full sample)

Corps	Sample Size	Number of Respondents	Response Rate (%)
Medical Corps	2,436	932	38.2
Nurse Corps	1,500	560	37.3
Medical Specialist Corps	500	177	35.4
Dental Corps	300	147	49.0
Veterinary Corps	200	102	51.0
Medical Service Corps	1,000	411	41.1
Enlisted Corps	2,000	281	14.1
Total	7,936	2,610	32.9

Figure 3.1
Conceptual Model of Deployment Experiences on Impact of PROFIS and Retention Intentions

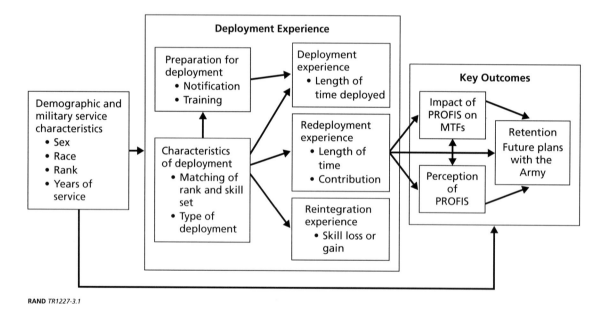

RAND *TR1227-3.1*

of contribution to the unit during redeployment); and the reintegration experience (whether clinical skills were perceived to have improved or degraded, how long it took to regain clinical skills if they degraded). We anticipated that health care professionals' deployment experiences would be affected by their demographic and military service characteristics, including their sex, race, marital status, number of dependents, AOC, rank, and years of active duty military service.

Weights

We calculated weights to account for differential sampling rates among strata and response rates by individual characteristics. To account for differential sampling rates, we formed design weights as the inverse of the probability of selection in a stratum. Survey respondents had more years on active duty and were of higher rank than nonrespondents (Tables 3.5 and 3.6). To account for differential response rates, we formed nonresponse weights as the inverse of the predicted probability of response among our sample, using models with predictors of rank, days since last deployment, and years on active duty. We formed final survey weights as the product of the design and nonresponse weights. We used the weights in analyses that combined strata for unadjusted analyses, and in regressions.

Missing Observations

With few exceptions, less than 3 percent of responses were missing for individual questions. Approximately 10 percent of responses were missing for questions related to the extent to which backfill is used, but these questions did not have "unknown" as a response option. We did not identify statistically significant relationships between missing data and descriptive variables, thus we assumed that the value that each individual would have selected is unrelated to the probability that the data are missing, given other variables. As such, we excluded observations from analyses if they had missing values for relevant variables that were not due to the skip patterns in the survey.

Descriptive Statistics

We produced and explored descriptive statistics for our variables of interest and examined differences in these measures by the deployment experience (e.g., number and duration of deployments, type of unit with which the provider deployed) and soldier characteristics (type

Table 3.5
Comparison of Responders to Nonresponders, by Corps: Rank

Corps/Responder Status		n	% E-1–E-4	% E-5	% E-6	% E-7–E-9	% O-1–O-4	% O-5–O-7	p-value*
Medical Corps	Responders	932	–	–	–	–	61.7	38.4	<0.0001
	Nonresponders	1,524	–	–	–	–	78.0	22.0	
Nurse Corps	Responders	560	–	–	–	–	81.7	18.3	<0.0001
	Nonresponders	940	–	–	–	–	89.5	10.5	
Medical Specialist Corps	Responders	177	–	–	–	–	88.5	11.5	0.0036
	Nonresponders	323	–	–	–	–	95.5	4.6	
Dental Corps	Responders	147	–	–	–	–	50.9	49.1	0.0001
	Nonresponders	153	–	–	–	–	72.7	27.3	
Veterinary Corps	Responders	102	–	–	–	–	63.4	36.6	0.0214
	Nonresponders	98	–	–	–	–	78.4	21.6	
Medical Service Corps	Responders	411	–	–	–	–	76.4	23.6	<0.0001
	Nonresponders	589	–	–	–	–	88.9	11.1	
Enlisted Corps	Responders	281	31.3	22.8	23.1	22.8	–	–	<0.0001
	Nonresponders	1,719	59.3	19.9	12.3	8.5	–	–	

NOTE: * p-value compares responders to nonresponders using chi-square tests.

Table 3.6
Comparison of Responders to Nonresponders, by Corps: Base Active Service Duty Years

Corps/Responder Status		n	Mean Base Active Service Duty Years (std)	p-value*
Medical Corps	Responders	932	10.5 (7.3)	<0.0001
	Nonresponders	1,524	7.6 (6.6)	
Nurse Corps	Responders	560	10.9 (7.6)	<0.0001
	Nonresponders	940	8.4 (7.3)	
Medical Specialist Corps	Responders	177	11.3 (7.1)	0.0588
	Nonresponders	323	13.3 (7.7)	
Dental Corps	Responders	147	12.4 (9.8)	0.0004
	Nonresponders	153	8.4 (8.6)	
Veterinary Corps	Responders	102	10.9 (8.1)	0.3301
	Nonresponders	98	8.1 (6.8)	
Medical Service Corps	Responders	411	11.0 (8.1)	0.0011
	Nonresponders	589	8.8 (7.0)	
Enlisted Corps	Responders	281	9.7 (6.6)	<0.0001
	Nonresponders	1,719	5.6 (5.7)	

NOTE: * p-value compares responders with nonresponders using t-tests.

of AMEDD corps, rank, years of service, etc.) using cross-tabulations and difference in means. Table 3.7 presents the demographic characteristics of the survey respondents, while Table 3.8 summarizes their service characteristics. For each of our three outcomes, we combined the two most positive response options, as well as the two least positive response options. For example, for the question "How equitable or fair is the PROFIS system overall?" we combine "very equitable" and "equitable." We also combined "very inequitable" and "inequitable" to facilitate interpretation of the analyses. "Neither equitable nor inequitable" was included as a response option. When analyzing factors associated with viewing PROFIS as inequitable, we combined "neither equitable nor inequitable" with "equitable." Analogously, when analyzing factors associated with viewing PROFIS as equitable, we combined "neither equitable nor inequitable" with "inequitable." We examined bivariate relationships between the demographic and military survey characteristics, the deployment characteristics, and the three outcomes. Selected results are presented in Chapter Four, with additional results from the survey provided in Appendix K.

Regressions

We performed logistic regression analyses to understand the relationships between demographic characteristics, deployment experiences, and the four outcomes of interest: (1) perceived skills degradation during deployment, (2) impact of PROFIS on the MTFs, (3) perception of PROFIS, and (4) retention (See Figure 3.1). To understand the impact of PROFIS on the MTFs, we examined the perception that workload increased or significantly increased among

Table 3.7
Demographic Characteristics of Responders

	Medical Corps	Nurse Corps	Medical Specialist Corps	Dental Corps	Veterinary Corps	Medical Service Corps	Enlisted Corps
N	932	560	177	147	102	411	281
Male (%)	81.4	36.5	69.3	83.0	51.0	71.1	67.3
Age (%)							
Under 30	10.6	24.1	17.7	10.9	18.6	25.0	45.2
30–34	20.0	11.1	17.1	18.4	11.8	12.2	15.7
35–39	26.4	17.1	18.9	10.2	17.6	22.2	17.1
40–44	17.7	18.7	24.0	12.9	15.7	20.6	13.5
45–49	14.3	16.9	14.3	14.3	18.6	14.1	7.1
50 and older	11.0	12.2	8.0	33.3	17.6	5.9	1.4
Race/ethnicity							
Black	3.5	14.5	3.4	8.8	3.9	15.5	18.1
White	82.6	67.3	84.7	68.7	87.3	69.6	59.4
Other	13.9	18.2	11.9	22.4	8.8	14.8	22.4
Hispanic	3.3	9.7	10.4	5.8	2.0	7.8	21.1
Marital status (%)							
Never married	11.0	20.5	14.7	9.5	21.6	13.2	12.8
Married	85.0	65.2	75.1	83.0	68.6	75.6	71.2
Separated	0.6	1.4	1.1	2.0	2.0	2.1	3.2
Divorced	3.3	12.2	8.5	4.8	7.9	8.9	12.8
Widowed	0.1	0.7	0.6	0.7	0.0	0.3	0.0
Any children in household (%)	60.4	49.0	53.8	59.1	46.7	55.6	50.3

those reporting that others had been deployed from their MTF. To understand the perception of PROFIS, we examined factors associated with the perception that overall PROFIS is inequitable or very inequitable. To understand retention, we examined the factors associated with the following dependent variables: (1) time away (or lack thereof) from their permanent duty station somewhat or strongly increased desire to leave and (2) unlikely to remain in the military for 20 years. Four sets of analyses were performed for (1) all respondents, (2) those who had been deployed, (3) the subset of deployed who were in PROFIS positions, and (4) those who reported that others had deployed from their MTF.

Each model had a different set of covariates relevant to the outcome of interest. Models controlled for demographics and service characteristics (rank, prior military experience, and corps). Skills degradation models were limited to those who have deployed and, in addition to covariates previously mentioned, included variables for whether the deployment lasted more

Table 3.8
Military Service Characteristics of Responders

	Medical Corps	Nurse Corps	Medical Specialist Corps	Dental Corps	Veterinary Corps	Medical Service Corps	Enlisted Corps
Rank							
E-1–E-4	–	–	–	–	–	–	31.3
E-5	–	–	–	–	–	–	22.8
E-6	–	–	–	–	–	–	23.1
E-7–E-9	–	–	–	–	–	–	22.8
O-1–O-4	59.4	81.8	88.1	47.7	63.7	74.4	–
O-5-O-9	40.6	18.2	11.7	52.4	36.3	25.6	–
Time on active duty							
1 year or less	6.2	11.5	6.3	15.3	15.8	11.0	6.5
2–5 years	19.9	20.5	14.8	22.2	16.8	19.2	28.3
6–10 years	26.2	16.8	19.3	11.1	22.8	18.4	26.1
11–15 years	18.5	18.3	17.6	10.4	17.8	15.0	14.5
16–20 years	16.4	21.4	18.2	11.8	13.9	19.1	18.8
21 or more years	12.8	11.4	23.9	29.2	12.9	17.3	5.8
Prior military service experience	28.9	48.6	67.8	22.8	31.3	45.7	33.3
Number of deployments 2001–2009							
0	32.8	34.6	18.1	51.0	49.0	27.2	29.9
1	39.1	41.6	32.8	36.7	29.4	36.8	37.0
2	17.2	17.1	22.0	8.2	16.7	25.6	20.3
3	6.0	5.4	16.4	2.7	3.9	5.1	9.6
4 or more	4.9	1.3	10.7	1.4	1.0	5.3	3.2
Current ADSO (2010)							
None (passed ADSO)	11.7	26.3	28.2	15.6	16.7	44.9	1.1
Less than 1 year	10.4	12.9	14.7	11.6	9.8	10.1	22.3
1–2 years (2011–2012)	26.0	25.9	24.9	27.2	26.5	18.4	10.4
3–4 years (2013–2014)	34.2	30.2	26.6	41.5	38.2	17.9	41.4
More than 5 years (2015 or later)	17.7	4.8	5.6	4.1	8.8	8.6	24.8

NOTE: ADSO = Active Duty Service Obligation.

than nine months and whether the person deployed in a PROFIS position. Models that included all officers had corps as covariates, while the model limited to the Medical Corps included covariates for strata and, for relevant strata, indicators for whether the individual deployed as a battalion surgeon. Models of perception of PROFIS included tier into which AOC fell, whether the person had been deployed (models that included all respondents), whether deployment had lasted more than nine months and whether deployed in a PROFIS position (models including just those who had deployed), frequency and satisfaction with communication with consultant (models that included officers), reported skill loss (models with officers who had deployed), timing of receipt of orders and satisfaction with integration into deploying unit (model that included officers who deployed in PROFIS position), and increased work hours as result of others deploying from MTF (model that included officers who reported others had deployed from their MTF). Retention models included covariates for tier into which AOC fell, whether the person had been deployed (models that included all respondents), whether deployment had lasted more than nine months and whether deployed in a PROFIS position (models including just those who had deployed), reported skill loss (models with officers who had deployed), increased work hours as result of others deploying from MTF (model that included officers who reported others had deployed from their MTF), and perception of PROFIS equity. Collinearity diagnostics were examined for each set of predictors. Chapter Four presents selected results, and Appendix L presents complete results.

Army Medical Department Resource Tasking System (ARTS) Data

We used ARTS data to conduct analyses on length of deployments and task/provider AOC/ MOS match. We acquired data on ARTS taskers to U.S. Central Command for medical personnel. The data contain information on all PROFIS deployments that began between September 12, 2001, and October 31, 2010, for both the tasking and the individual filling the tasking. Information on the tasking included the tasking number, position number, the task AOC/MOS, and the purpose of the tasking (PROFIS, PROFIS Replacement, Medical Augmentation, Medical Augmentation Replacement, Backfill, Admin, Active Component/ Reserve Component, and Active Component/Reserve Component Bridge), the tasking mission (OIF, OEF, Operation New Dawn), the deploying unit, and the beginning date and end date for the deployment. Future and ongoing deployments have an estimated end date, which is updated upon redeployment. Information about the person filling the tasking included the person's primary AOC/MOS, ASIs, the providing regional medical command, the providing unit, and the person's rank.

The data include information on 11,814 PROFIS deployments. Of these, 80.4 percent were to OIF, 15.6 percent were to OEF, and 4.0 percent were in support of other missions, including Operation New Dawn, research, training, and humanitarian assistance. Some 2,386 records (20.2 percent) are missing provider AOC/MOS. Discussion with AMEDD indicated that these missing data are due to mis-merging of files caused by data entry errors. Missing AOCs/MOSs were more common in 2002 through 2004 than in later years, and more common among more junior ranks, suggesting that data quality improved over time and that data errors frequently were identified and corrected the longer someone was in the Army. The extent to which AOCs/MOSs were missing varied by corps; missing data were more common in the Nurse Corps and Enlisted Corps.

We analyzed deployment information for the Medical, Nurse, Dental, Veterinary, Medical Service, Medical Specialist, and Enlisted Corps. We focused analyses on deployments that were at least 30 days in duration to exclude short-term deployments—for example, those that were for the purpose of obtaining information for longer deployments.

Length of deployment was determined by subtracting the deployment start date from the deployment end date. For the length of deployment analyses, we excluded deployments beginning in 2010 because the return date had not been observed for many of them.

For the analyses of task/provider AOC/MOS match, the research team restricted the analyses to records not missing provider AOC/MOS and included all PROFIS deployments, regardless of whether the health care professional was still deployed. We used substitutability criteria (AR 601-142, 2007, Table 1) to characterize the skills match between the provider and the requirement of the tasking. In some cases, AMEDD uses not only the AOC/MOS of the tasking and health care professional, but also additional skills designated by the ASI in the determination of whether a health care professional is suitable for a task. While the ASI of the provider was available in the data, the ASI of the tasking was not; therefore, we considered only AOC/MOS in the determination of task/provider AOC/MOS match. The ARTS data contain only the primary AOC/MOS of the provider; it is possible that in some cases a secondary AOC/MOS would indicate a match or approved substitution where the primary AOC/MOS indicates a non-approved substitution.

We placed deployments into one of four categories:

1. **Field positions**, which can be filled by numerous health care professional AOCs, included deployments where the AOC of the tasking was either 60A (operational medicine), 62B (field surgeon), 61N (flight surgeon), 63R (executive dentist), or 64Z (senior veterinarian).
2. **Matched positions**, where the provider and the tasking have the same AOC/MOS and the tasking AOC is not one of the field positions above. For the Medical Service Corps, we counted medical functional areas and the corresponding AOCs as a match.
3. **Approved substitution**, where the provider AOC/MOS is approved to substitute for the task AOC/MOS. Providers with an AOC of 60Q (pediatric subspecialist) were considered approved substitutes for the same AOCs as 60P (pediatrician),[3] which is consistent with MEDCOM practices.
4. **Non-approved substitutions**, where none of the above conditions were met. We further analyzed the subset of Medical Corps field position deployments. We analyzed these deployments by categorizing the provider's AOC in two ways: (1) the strata created for the survey and (2) the substitution groups for these field positions listed in AR 601-142.

Administrative Data

For analyses of deployments (both organic and PROFIS) and retention during OEF/OIF, we used four administrative datasets that track personnel: the Active Duty Military Pay File, Reserve Pay File, Work Experience File, and Proxy Personnel Tempo. These files are maintained by the Defense Manpower Personnel Data Center (DMDC), which is responsible for all Department of Defense personnel data. We used October 2001 through December 2009 data for active duty Army personnel who had an AOC/MOS for one of AMEDD's corps at some point during the time period. The datasets are linked using a scrambled identifier,

---

[3]   60Q did not exist when regulation was written; delineated as 60P or 60P with specialist training.

enabling the creation of a file that tracks AMEDD personnel on a monthly basis from October 2001 or the month they enter the data (whichever is later) until they leave active duty Army or December 2009 (whichever is earlier).

The analytic file includes information and tracks changes over time in demographics and family characteristics, rank, the person's primary duty AOC/MOS, up to two ASIs/skill identfiers, unit, base pay, receipt of hazardous duty pay (which is used to identify deployments), and receipt of additional special pay (e.g., retention bonuses). We identified when individuals were in an internship, residency, or a training unit.[4] In addition to tracking the person's career from 2001 to 2009, the data also include information on when the service member joined the military, years of service, and when their current service obligation will be or was completed (for those who completed their service obligation during the time examined). This information was missing for individuals who completed their service obligation before the start of the data period being examined. While the data contain a variable for duty AOC/MOS, we determined that the quality of these data was not sufficient to be able to identify when a person was deployed outside his or her specialty (e.g., when a specialist was deployed in a field surgeon position).

Administrative Data Analyses

We used the administrative data to analyze **deployments** and **retention** in the military after completion of service obligations.

Deployment

We defined deployment as receiving hostile fire pay for at least two consecutive months. This definition was adopted to exclude short-term deployments, such as those by unit leadership that were for the purpose of preparing for longer deployments. These analyses include all deployments; we were not able to distinguish between organic and PROFIS deployments in the data. We also could not distinguish between when someone was selected for deployment versus when someone volunteered for deployment. We restricted our analyses to those individuals for whom we observed at least six months of consecutive data outside of training. All analyses were conducted separately for each corps.

We conducted a series of analyses to understand how the burden of deployment may vary by corps, AOC/MOS, and individual characteristics.[5] We calculated for each quarter the percentage of person-months that individuals were deployed, by corps, strata, and AOC/MOS. We excluded providers identified as being in training that quarter, because they are not considered eligible to deploy by MEDCOM until their training is completed. However, we were not able to identify people who are not deployable for other reasons, such as profiles.

We calculated descriptive statistics on the percentage of people who were in the Army in December 2009 who were deployed zero times, once, twice, and three or more times between October 2001 and the end of 2009. We required personnel to be in a nontraining unit for at least six consecutive months to be included in these analyses. To assess factors associated with deployment, we estimated corps-specific logistic regression models using person-level data for

---

[4]   We could not identify when physicians or other providers were in a fellowship program unless they were in a training unit. Based on discussions with AMEDD personnel, the way in which training units are used and assigned depends on the specific MTF.

[5]   We used corps-specific models to improve the interpretability of the models and avoid excessive use of interaction terms.

those still in the Army at the end of 2009. The first model estimated being deployed at least once as a function of demographic characteristics (age in 2009, sex, race, marital status in 2009, change in marital status since person was first observed in data, having at least one dependent child in 2009, and increase in the number of dependent children since the person was first observed in data) and service characteristics (including AOC/strata in 2009, change in AOC/strata since the person was first observed in the data, years of service, rank in 2009, and indicators for the years the person was not a trainee during the timeframe of the data). We included interaction terms between indicators for years of duty not in training and selected AOCs and demographic characteristics to improve model fit in corps where diagnostic plots suggested they might be useful.

We developed a second model assessing factors associated with multiple deployments among those deployed at least once, using the same covariates just described. We also developed a third model assessing factors associated with more than two deployments among those deployed at least twice, using a subset of covariates from the other deployment models. Due to the small number of multiple deployments within Veterinary Corps and Dental Corps, we did not construct the third model for these corps. Within each corps, we used results of the three models to predict the probability that each person deploys zero, one, two, and three or more times for everyone in the corps, using recycled predictions using a standardized set of demographic characteristics and years of military service across corps.[6] These facilitate the interpretation of differences between deployment histories of different groups that are easier to interpret than the model coefficients, but, like coefficients, are adjusted for all other predictors in the model. We also performed recycled predictions for gender, race, and AOC/MOS/stratum.[7] The results of these analyses are summarized in Chapter Four, and complete regression results are presented in Appendix M.

Retention

We used different approaches for modeling the effect of deployment on retention in the Army for the enlisted and officer corps. Enlisted soldiers make a decision to leave or stay in the Army at their expiration of term of service (ETS) date, even if the decision is to extend their contract for some amount of time without formally reenlisting. Officers, however, can remain in the military after the end of their service obligation without making a commitment to spending a specific amount of additional time in the Army.

For the enlisted corps, we modeled the first reenlistment decision. We restricted the sample to those with a pay entry base date of January 2000 or later and whose initial ETS date was before the end of 2009, to ensure that we would observe the first time they faced a reenlistment

---

[6]   p(1+) was given by the first model.
  p(3+ given deployed) was given by the third model.
  p(0) = 1 − p(1+)
  p(1) = p(1+) × (1 − p(2+ given deployed))
  p(2) = p(2+) × (1 − p(3+ given deployed 2+))
  p(3+) = p(2+) × p(3+ given deployed 2+)
  p(0) + p(1) + p(2) + p(3+) summed to 100 percent for each person.

[7]   For each characteristic for which we did adjusted probabilities, (male, female, each AOC, etc.), we estimated the probability of having deployed zero, one, two, or three or more times, if everyone in the corps had that characteristic. We then took the average of all the predicted probabilities for zero, one, two, and three or more within the corps for that characteristic.

decision.[8] We excluded those individuals who served less than three years before leaving the Army and those who left the Army six months or more before their ETS date. We inferred reenlistment decisions by examining monthly information about the ETS time remaining (Hosek and Totten, 2002; Hosek and Martorell, 2009). We assumed that the first time the ETS date increased by at least two years was their first reenlistment decision. If an individual left active duty before the last month of the data and before their ETS date increased by at least two years, we assumed that they left the Army rather than reenlisting. Consistent with the approach developed by Hosek and Martorell (2009), we assumed that people whose ETS increased by less than 24 months had extended their contract. These were not considered to be reenlistment or exit decisions. Individuals extending their contracts by less than 24 months were followed until their ETS date increased by at least 24 months, they exited the Army, or the end of our data, at which point we could no longer observe their decisions. Toward the end of the period covered by our data, some of the individuals who extended were not observed to separate or increase their ETS by 24 months or more; these individuals are excluded from the analysis.

Our main predictors of interest are the number of deployments or cumulative months of deployment before the first reenlistment decision. Consistent with the approach developed by Hosek and Martorell (2009), we included in our counts only deployments that ended more than three months before a reenlistment decision was made, because the favorable tax implications of reenlisting while deployed would create an upward-biased estimate of the effect of deployment on reenlistment.

We ran both logistic and linear probability models of deciding to reenlist. The results were similar. The coefficients for the linear model are more easily interpreted; therefore, we present those results in the next chapter. Covariates measured at the time of reenlistment decisions that were included in the model are demographic characteristics (gender, race, age, marital status, and number of dependent children), service characteristics (length of service, grade, and MOS), the availability and size of selective reenlistment bonuses[9] for the person's MOS in the quarter of the reenlistment decision, calendar year, and either the number of deployments or cumulative months of deployments before the first reenlistment decision. We included interaction terms between the number of deployments and the year the decision was made, as we suspected that the effect of deployments on reenlistment might change over time.

For the officer corps, we developed corps-specific discrete time duration models for the time to leaving active duty. We adopted this approach because, as mentioned, officers can remain in the Army after the completion of their service obligation without making a specific commitment, and it is difficult in the administrative data to distinguish between increases in commitment due to decisions to stay in the military from decisions to obtain additional training. To focus our analyses on the time after individual's first ADSO, we restricted the analysis to those individuals who entered the Army either after October 2001 or within three years prior to October 2001 (i.e., after October 1998). For those individuals who entered the Army prior to October 2001, time at risk of leaving active duty was defined as beginning on the month of their ADSO date in October 2001. For those individuals observed entering the

---

[8]   The analyses excluded individuals who moved from the enlisted corps to the officer corps prior to their ETS date.

[9]   We do not interpret the coefficient for the bonus variable, as bonuses are used only when attrition is deemed problematic for an AOC.

Army after October 2001, time at risk began in the month of their first ADSO date.[10] Each person was either observed to leave or, if they were in the data on the last month of the data (December 2009), their time at risk was censored.

We used a complementary log-log link between the predicted probability of leaving active duty and the linear prediction from the model. In this form, exponentiation of the coefficients gives a hazard ratio: the risk of leaving the Army for those with the characteristic divided by the risk for baseline group (for categorical predictors) among those who have not yet left active duty. We modeled the baseline risk nonparametrically. Each person was at risk for up to eight years and three months (the longest observed time would be for someone who was past their ADSO date in October 2001 and remained in the Army through December 2009). Each year of time at risk had its own baseline hazard; in order to support baseline estimation with dwindling numbers of observations, we assumed the last three years to have a constant hazard. Those who were observed in the data in October 2001 and those observed to enter the data after October 2001 had a separate baseline hazard over time.

Our predictor of interest was deployment history. We included both deployment before time at risk started (time-invariant) and deployment after risk started (time-varying). We do not, however, interpret the coefficients for deployments after risk started, as this is endogenous with retention.[11] We characterized deployment history both as number of times deployed and cumulative months of deployment.[12] Covariates included in the model are demographic characteristics (gender, race, age, marital status, and number of dependent children), service characteristics (length of service, rank and AOC/stratum), the average size of bonuses for the person's AOC (officer special pay bonus, a medical officer incentive pay bonus, medical special pay, or nurse bonus that quarter in that AOC), indicator variables for being a trainee or being deployed (both of which reduced the likelihood of leaving the Army that month), and the calendar year the person became at risk for leaving the Army. Many of the covariates were allowed to vary over time. For each officer corps, we used results of the models to generate recycled predictions for the probability of remaining on active duty over time if we varied the cumulative months deployed before the end of their service obligation. These facilitate the interpretation of the effect of deployment history on retention in the military in that they are easier to interpret than the model coefficients, but, like coefficients, are adjusted for all other predictors in the model. The results of these analyses are summarized in Chapter Four, and complete regression results are presented in Appendix N.

---

[10] Based on our analyses, it appeared that the first observed ADSO date included service obligations incurred during military residency training.

[11] Even if deployment after risk started increased someone's interest in leaving the Army, it would reduce the person's ability to actually do so, as the person would not be able to voluntarily leave active duty while deployed.

[12] As mentioned previously, we were unable to distinguish when someone was selected for a deployment versus when someone volunteered for a deployment. The relationship between voluntary deployments and retention may be very different than the relationship between other deployments and retention.

CHAPTER FOUR

Effect of and Concerns About PROFIS

Following our initial interviews with stakeholders and MEDCOM and FORSCOM staff, we developed a list of key issues and concerns regarding PROFIS. These issues vary in importance and degree by stakeholder. Our survey, follow-on interviews, and other data analysis plans were designed to inform these issues. This chapter presents these issues and concerns and the supporting evidence for them.

Stakeholders and Issues

Using what we learned in the interviews, we grouped stakeholders into four categories: health care professionals; MTF and regional medical command commanders, managers, and administrative staff; Office of the Surgeon General/MEDCOM staff; and receiving (deploying) unit commanders and staff. Many health care professionals have concerns about how PROFIS affects their medical skills, career, and family. Some MTF and regional medical command personnel have these concerns as well but also worry about how to fill slots in PROFIS and how well the system works. Office of the Surgeon General/MEDCOM stakeholders are concerned with many of the same issues but must also implement PROFIS and interact with the receiving unit commands. Finally, receiving unit stakeholders often have very different perspectives and issues with regard to their PROFIS personnel and the system as a whole, including how PROFIS personnel integrate into the unit and how prepared they are for deployment.

We identified five categories of issues and concerns: equity, predictability, skills and training, impact on the MTFs, and retention (Table 4.1).

Briefly, **equity** refers to the overall sense of fairness of the system (e.g., how often one group of individuals deploys as compared with another) as well as individual issues related to equity, such as type and length of deployments. In this category, we also describe issues pertaining to one specific position, the battalion surgeon, which generates equity concerns within the Medical Corps and is an important position for receiving units.

Predictability refers to the reported short notice of deployments from the standpoint of the health care professionals, managers of the system, and the receiving unit. For the receiving units, the issue is that the PROFIS personnel designated to join the unit can change frequently, even very close to the unit deployment date.

The **skills and training** category refers to both the clinical and surgical skills that health care professionals bring and apply in their PROFIS assignments, the soldier and leadership skills/training they need while deployed, and the effect deployment has on these skills.

Table 4.1
Issues About PROFIS, by Stakeholder

Issue Category	Issues	Primary Stakeholders
Equity	Who is deploying	Health care professionals
	Number of times individuals deploy	Health care professionals/MTFs/ regional medical command
	Length of deployments	Health care professionals/receiving units
	Type of deployments	Health care professionals
	Battalion surgeon positions	Health care professionals/receiving units
Predictability	Short notice of deployment	Health care professionals/MTFs/ regional medical command/ Office of the Surgeon General
	Health care professional assigned to PROFIS position keeps changing	Receiving units
Skills and training	Skills mismatch	Health care professionals/receiving units
	Underutilization/low caseload in specialty	Health care professionals/MTFs
Impact on MTFs	Increased workload	Health care professionals/MTFs
	Perception of reduced access	Health care professionals/MTFs
Retention	Impact of deployments on retention and intention to remain in military	Health care professionals/MTFs/ Office of the Surgeon General

Impact on the MTFs includes perceptions of the workload on the remaining staff and the ability of MTFs to backfill for deployed personnel, as well as the potential appearance of reduced access to care at the MTFs.

Finally, **retention** addresses the effect of deployments and PROFIS on retention intentions of health care professionals.

The rest of this chapter describes each of these issues in more detail, drawing on our interview data, the survey, and deployment and other data to quantify and, potentially, confirm or deny the validity of these concerns. We report some results at the AMEDD level, some at the corps level (Medical Corps, Nurse Corps, Medical Specialist Corps, Dental Corps, Veterinary Corps, Medical Service Corps, Enlisted Corps), and a few at the AOC or groups of AOC level. For more detailed data describing individual AOCs and groups of AOCs within a corps, please see Appendixes C, D, E, F, G, H, and I.

Equity of Deployments

Equity encompasses a variety of factors, the importance of which varies by stakeholder. Generally, when we talked to PROFIS personnel, the equity issues that they described were in terms of the length of deployments, the number of deployments, and the types of positions they were being sent to, including, in the Medical Corps, the battalion surgeon position.

As part of our analysis of equity, we calculated the percentage of person-months that personnel were deployed in each quarter from 2002 to 2009 for all corps. These data include personnel who deploy as PROFIS providers as well as personnel who deploy in organic positions (e.g., personnel permanently assigned in TDA or TOE units). Overall, after a sharp peak followed by a drop in 2003 at the start of OIF, the percentage has increased slightly through 2009 for all corps (Figure 4.1). The Medical Specialist Corps consistently has the highest percentage of personnel deployed, followed by the Enlisted Corps and Medical Service Corps. The Medical Corps and Nurse Corps are next in terms of percentage deployed. The Veterinary Corps and Dental Corps have the lowest percentage of personnel deployed during most quarters over the past eight years.

However, looking at deployment by corps masks the variability that exists within a corps. Personnel in some AOCs are more likely to be deployed than others. Figure 4.2 shows the seven AOCs (and groups of AOCs) with the highest percentage of personnel-time deployed and the five AOCs with the lowest number of personnel-time deployed.

In the top seven, five corps are represented: physician assistants (65D) are the most likely to be deployed, followed by health care specialists (combat medics) (68W), and then general surgeons (61J), family medicine physicians and their substitutes,[1] nurse anesthetists (66F), health care administrators (67A and 70 series[2]) and behavioral sciences, social work, and clinical psychologists (67D, 73A and 73B). Similarly, three different corps are represented in the

Figure 4.1
Percentage of Personnel-Time Deployed, by Corps and Quarter (PROFIS and Organic)

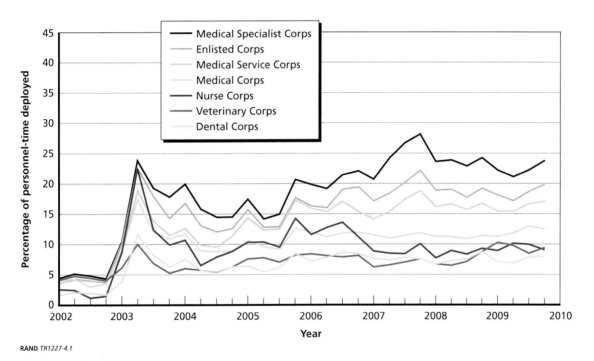

___

[1] Family medicine physicians and their substitutions include family physicians (61H), pediatricians (60P), emergency physicians (62A), internists (61F), flight surgeons (61N), and field surgeons (62B).

[2] The 70 series includes health care administrator (70A), health services administration (70B), health services comptroller (70C), health services systems manager (IMO) (70D), patient administrator (70E), health services human resource manager (70F), health services plans, operations, intelligence, security, and training (70H), and health services materiel officer (70K).

Figure 4.2
Highest and Lowest Percentages of Personnel-Time Deployed, by Quarter (PROFIS and Organic)

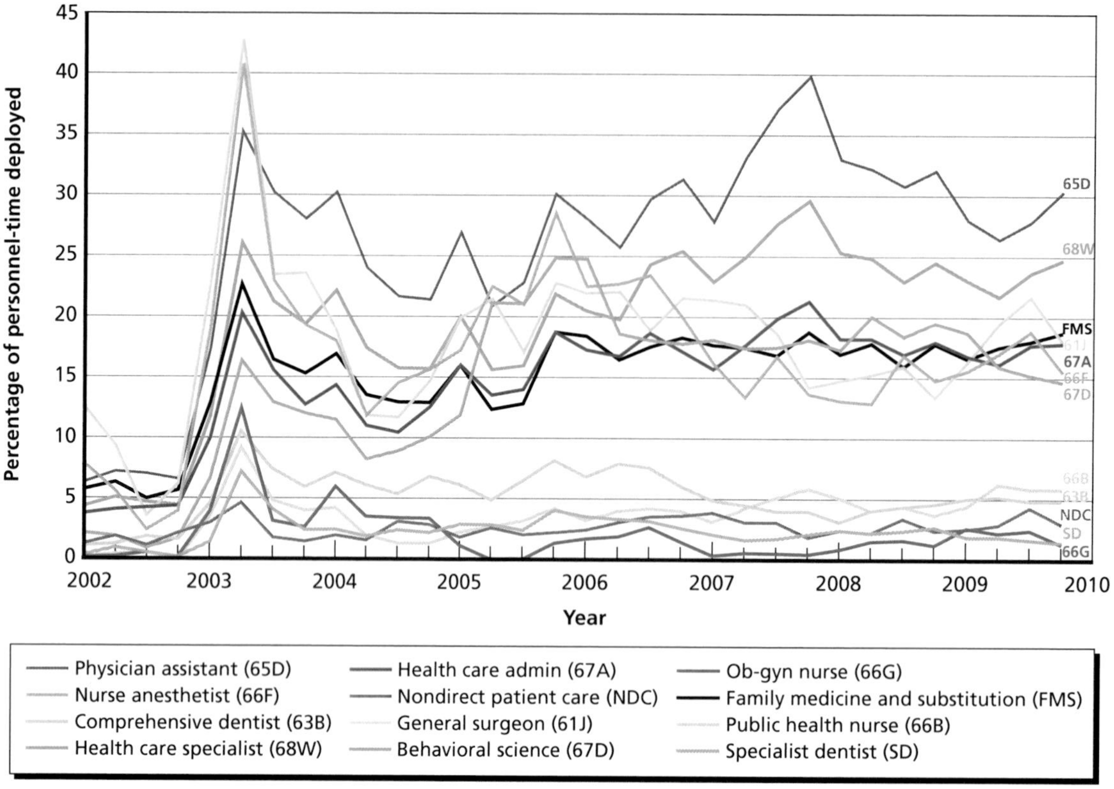

RAND TR1227-4.2

bottom five deploying groups: public health (66B) and OB/GYN (66G) nurses, all dentists except general and comprehensive dentists,[3] and physicians not involved in direct patient care.[4]

The percentage of personnel-time deployed is one measure of equity; however, this metric does not capture the frequency or length of deployments for individuals. We also analyzed the history of deployments by individual for those personnel in the active duty Army in December 2009, controlling for demographic and service characteristics (Figure 4.3). For personnel to be included in these data, they had to be available for deployment (e.g., not in a training unit, not a resident, and not an intern) for at least six months. The percentage of personnel who have never deployed ranges from 60 percent in the Veterinary Corps to only 26 percent in the Medical Specialist Corps. The Medical Specialist Corps has the highest percentage of repeat deployers, at 36 percent. Again, the corps-level data mask some of the within-corps variability. For instance, in most AOCs, less than 10 percent of current personnel have deployed two or more times. However, at least 20 percent of a small group of AOCs have deployed more than twice: physician assistants (53 percent), nurse anesthetists (51 percent), general surgeons (46 percent),

---

[3] This includes comprehensive dentists (63B), periodontists (63D), endodontists (63E), prosthodontists (63F), public health dentists (63H), pediatric dentists (63K), orthodontists (63M), oral and maxillofacial surgeons (63N), oral pathologists (63P), and executive dentists (63R).

[4] Nondirect patient care specialties are defined for this report as diagnostic radiologist (61R), therapeutic radiologist (61Q), and pathologist (61U).

Figure 4.3
Number of Deployments (PROFIS and Organic) per Individual, by Corps, for Personnel in the Army in December 2009

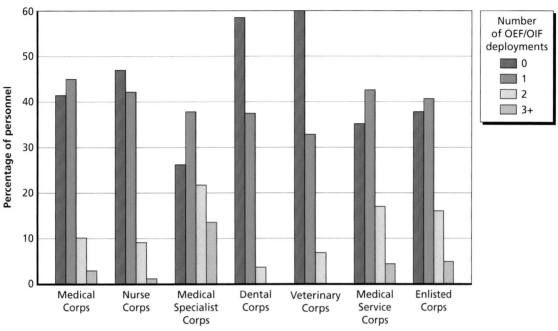

RAND *TR1227-4.3*

health care specialists (28 percent), health care administrators (24 percent), and other Medical Corps specialties[5] (21 percent). These data do not allow us to identify personnel who may have volunteered to deploy multiple times. For instance, Dental Corps leaders reported that only dentists who volunteered deployed more than once. However, based on our interview with health care professionals, we conjecture that it is unlikely that the majority of repeat deployers in other corps are volunteers.

In our interviews, some of the people who make the decisions about who is deployed (consultants, MTF staff and commanders, etc.) told us that they take into consideration personal situations in a way that could result in some groups being deployed more than others or having a higher likelihood of deploying than others. Therefore, we analyzed corps-specific data to try to determine whether there were any groups of personnel who were systematically being deployed more than others. These corps-specific multivariate analyses using personnel data showed significant associations between demographic characteristics and having been deployed at least once between October 2001 and December 2009 (Table 4.2), controlling for AOC, years of service, age, and number of years not in training during the time period examined (i.e., time at risk for deployment). Within-corps AOC results are reported in the corps-specific appendixes. In all corps, females were significantly less likely to have deployed than males. This can be explained in part, but probably not completely, by the fact that some combat positions are male-only. In addition, across some corps, blacks (Nurse Corps, Medical Service Corps, Enlisted Corps) and Hispanics (Nurse Corps) were less likely to have deployed

---

[5] Other Medical Corps specialties include operational medicine (60A), occupational medicine (60D), and preventive medicine (60C)

Table 4.2
Adjusted Probability of Deployment, by Demographics and Service Characteristics, with at Least One Deployment Among Active-Duty Personnel in December 2009 (%)

Characteristic	Medical Corps	Nurse Corps	Medical Specialist Corps	Dental Corps	Veterinary Corps	Medical Service Corps	Enlisted Corps
Gender							
Male (ref)	60.8	56.5	78.6	43.2	49.2	65.2	65.6
Female	50.2***	51.0**	66.5***	33.3*	29.3***	57.3***	53.3***
Race							
White (ref)	59.7	56.2	73.5	43.1	41.5	66.0	63.3
Black	58.8	44.6***	71.7			61.6*	58.9***
Hispanic	58.5	49.8*	77.7			63.5	63.5
Other[a]				37.0	30.4		
Marital status							
Never married (ref)	60.4	55.8	77.0	42.9	53.9	61.8	62.1
Married	58.6	51.6	72.6	40.8	34.7**	65.9	62.3
Became divorced							
No (ref)	58.4	52.8	73.8	41.4	40.1	63.9	61.6
Yes	60.5	53.7	70.9	39.7	37.6	76.5*	67.7***
Dependent child in December 2009							
No (ref)	60.1	55.3	75.2	42.8	39.3	67.2	63.6
Yes	57.7	51.2*	72.6	40.4	40.6	62.4*	60.7***
Officer rank							
Lower (ref)[b]	59.5	55.1	75.9	45.8	40.4	67.8	
Higher	53.4	43.9***	58.1***	31.6*	35.5	51.0***	
Enlisted rank							
E-1 to E-4 (ref)							58.0
E-5 to E-6							67.6***
E-7 and higher							65.8***

NOTES: * indicates p ≤ 0.05, ** indicates p ≤ 0.01, and *** indicates p ≤ 0.001. Analyses control for age, AOC/stratum in 2009, change in AOC/stratum since the person was first observed in the data, years of service, and amount of time in service not as a trainee.

[a] For groups with fewer observations, blacks, Hispanics, Asian/Pacific Islanders, and American Indians/Alaskan Natives were collapsed into the Other category.

[b] "Higher" rank for all groups except the Medical Corps, Dental Corps, and Veterinary Corps includes O-5 and above compared to O-1 to O-4. For the Veterinary Corps, Dental Corps, and Medical Corps, higher rank includes O-6 and above, compared with O-1 to O-5.

than non-Hispanic whites. It is not clear why this would be the case. Individuals in some, but not all, corps were significantly less likely to have deployed if they had dependent children. However, just being married was not protective of being deployed, except in the Veterinary Corps. This could indicate that some of the leaders making deployment assignments are considering family circumstances when choosing individuals to deploy. Higher-ranking officers in most officer corps[6] were significantly less likely to have deployed than lower-ranking officers, which confirms our interview data that fewer higher-ranking officers were deploying. However, higher-ranking enlisted personnel (E-5 and above) were more likely to deploy than E-4 and below, which is not surprising given that enlisted personnel are in training for the early parts of their service time.

We also analyzed characteristics associated with multiple deployments among those who deployed at least once (data not shown). Controlling for other factors, females in the Nurse Corps, Medical Corps, Medical Service Corps, Enlisted Corps, and Medical Specialist Corps were significantly less likely than males to deploy multiple times. Only in the Nurse Corps was having at least one dependent child associated with not deploying more than once, among those who had deployed. In the Medical Corps, being of higher rank (O-6 and above) was associated with not deploying more than once. Enlisted personnel were also less likely to deploy multiple times if they were black, Asian/Pacific Islander, or had a dependent child. E-5 or E-6 (compared with E-1 to E-4) were more likely to have multiple deployments. In the Medical Specialist Corps, Hispanics were significantly more likely to deploy more than one time. In the Medical Service Corps, married individuals were less likely to deploy twice.

Length of deployment is also not the same for all corps. These data vary by year because policy decisions made over the past ten years have changed the length of some PROFIS deployments, as described in Chapter Two. However, generally, units deploy for 12 months (with some exceptions), and health care professionals either deploy for the full time or, when applicable, split a full deployment near the six-month point. Thus, the distribution of deployment lengths has two peaks, at six and 12 months, with a dip at nine months, because actual lengths of deployment can vary, even for individuals who were sent for one-half of a deployment. Therefore, we analyzed the PROFIS deployments based on whether they were less than nine months or greater than or equal to nine months. In 2009, the last year for which we have complete data, the Enlisted and Medical Services Corps had a higher percentage of personnel who deployed for more than nine months, while the Nurse and Dental Corps had the fewest personnel (less than 25 percent) who deployed for more than nine months (Figure 4.4).

These deployment data highlight some of the concerns regarding equity in terms of frequency of deployments and length of deployments. However, perceptions of equity include other issues as well. In our survey, we asked personnel how equitable the PROFIS is overall. While some personnel reported that PROFIS was inequitable, they were the minority of respondents (Figure 4.5). In all corps, a large number of personnel (25–45 percent) reported that they do not know whether the system is equitable. The Medical Corps had the largest percentage (35 percent) of personnel who reported that PROFIS is inequitable. Factors associated with viewing PROFIS as inequitable from the multivariate analysis include[7]

---

[6]   For the Nurse Corps, Medical Specialist Corps, and Medical Service Corps, higher rank is O-5 and above for most recent rank observed; for the Dental Corps, higher rank is O-6 and above.

[7]   For complete results including odds ratios and p values see Appendix L.

Figure 4.4
Percentage of PROFIS Deployments Starting in 2009 That Were Less Than or Equal to Nine Months or Greater Than Nine Months in Duration, by Corps

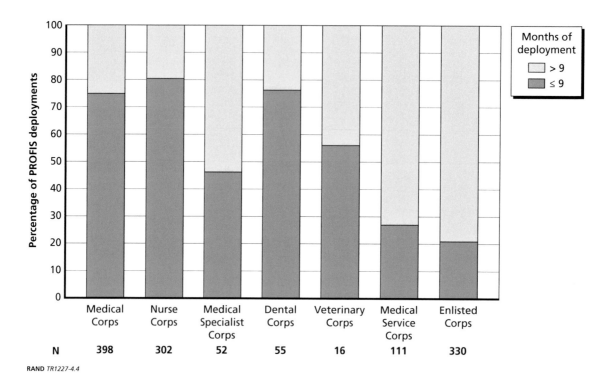

RAND TR1227-4.4

Figure 4.5
Views of Personnel on Equity of PROFIS

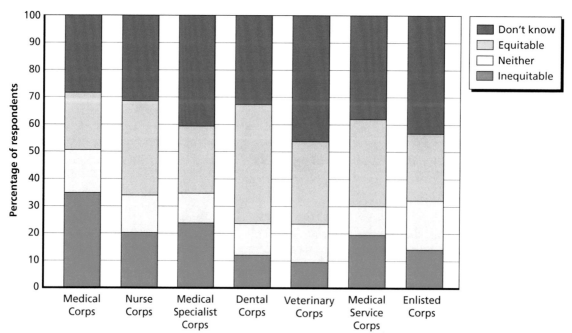

RAND TR1227-4.5

- deployment—whether the person had previously deployed as a PROFIS provider and number of deployments
- dissatisfaction with communication with their AOC consultant
- reporting experiencing skill loss while deployed
- dissatisfaction with integration into the unit in which they deployed as a PROFIS filler
- work hours increasing as a result of others deploying from their permanent duty station
- deployment as a battalion surgeon (Medical Corps only).

These indicate that issues other than just deployment length and frequency are important in terms of health care professionals' views of PROFIS.

Battalion Surgeon Positions

Part of the disparity between the Medical Corps and the other corps regarding the equity of PROFIS is due to the battalion surgeon position (62B). Contrary to the name, battalion surgeons are typically generalist or primary care physicians: family physicians, internists, pediatricians, or emergency medicine physicians. However, AR 601-142 stipulates that a number of other physician specialties can substitute as battalion surgeons (see Appendix J for full table of substitutability). From 2002 to 2010, 32 percent of battalion surgeon deployments were filled with other specialists (Figure 4.6).[8]

The job of a battalion surgeon can vary but typically includes sick call, some light trauma care, and acting as part of the leadership team in a battalion, providing medical advice and knowledge to that team. In garrison, the battalion physician assistant fills the role of the battalion surgeon, but, upon deployment, a PROFIS physician typically assumes that role. In our interviews, MEDCOM staff, regional medical command and MTF staff, and physicians themselves told us that this position creates a substantial amount of concern, especially since approximately one-third of all Medical Corps PROFIS deployments are in battalion surgeon positions.

In our survey, physicians who deploy as battalion surgeons were more likely to report that PROFIS is inequitable compared with the other physicians who could deploy as battalion surgeons but deploy in other positions (Figure 4.7). Battalion surgeon deployments are, on average, longer than most other PROFIS deployments for physicians (Figure 4.8). Physicians filling these roles were also more likely to report not being well prepared for the clinical duties while deployed (Figure 4.9) and that their skills degraded during deployment (Figure 4.10). Also, these positions often require a male physician because of combat exclusion restrictions on women, which adds to concerns about gender equity for deployment. From the receiving unit point of view, the battalion surgeon positions are important: Commanders want their batallion surgeon to train extensively with the unit prior to deployment; they prefer to have one batallion surgeon for the entire deployment; and, in some cases, they want their batallion surgeon to remain with the unit for 90 days following deployment to provide continuity of care for returning soldiers (ALARACT 306/2009, 2009). These demands create an added burden for

---

[8]   AR 601-142 lists approved substitutions for specific AOCs. However, the regulation needs to be updated to reflect current practices including allowing pediatric subspecialists, infectious disease physicians, and others to deploy in 62B positions.

Figure 4.6
Physicians Filling Battalion Surgeon Deployments (2002–2010)

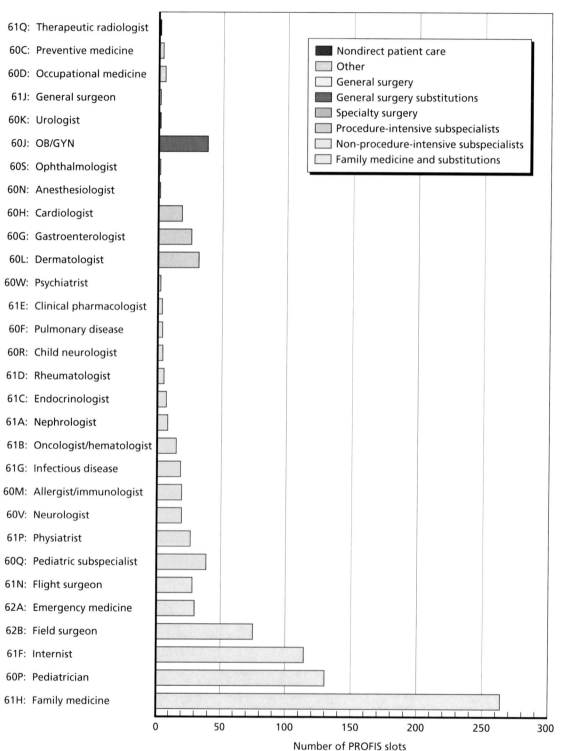

Figure 4.7
Views on PROFIS Equity Among Physicians Able to Deploy as Battalion Surgeons, by Whether They Deployed as Battalion Surgeons or in Other Positions

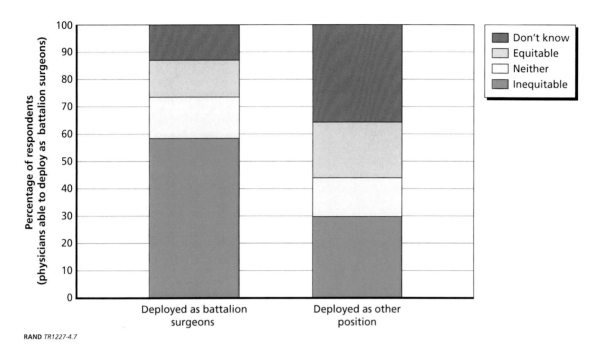

RAND *TR1227-4.7*

Figure 4.8
Among Physicians Able to Deploy as Battalion Surgeons, the Average Length of Deployments, by Deployment Type

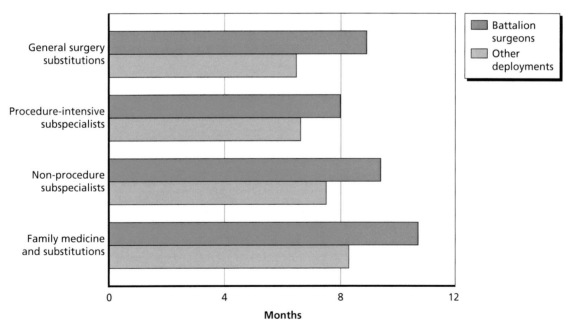

RAND *TR1227-4.8*

Figure 4.9
Extent to Which Physicians Able to Fill Battalion Surgeon Positions Felt Clinically Prepared When Deployed as Battalion Surgeons, Compared with Other Deployments, by Type of Specialty

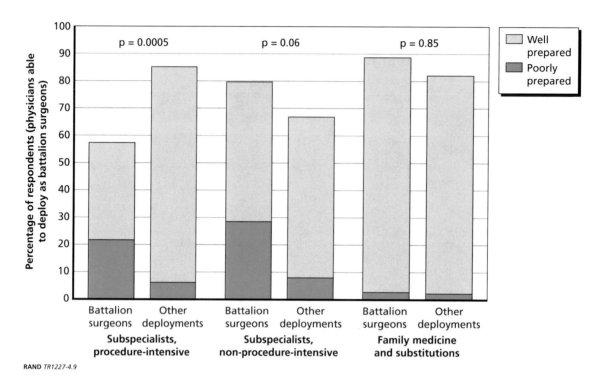

RAND *TR1227-4.9*

Figure 4.10
Extent to Which Physicians Able to Fill Battalion Surgeon Positions Report Experiencing Skill Degradation While Deployed as Battalion Surgeons, Compared with Other Deployments, by Type of Specialty

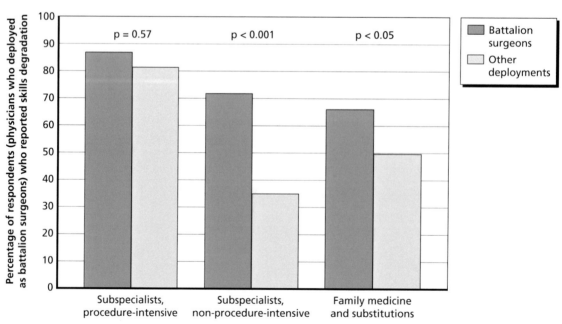

RAND *TR1227-4.10*

the physician, who is usually not from the same base as the deploying unit and must stay away from his or her home station for up to another 90 days.

Predictability

All stakeholders involved with PROFIS agree that it is better to identify PROFIS fillers early enough to enable them to become acquainted with their deploying units through adequate training opportunities. However, the current system does not achieve this goal. Ideally, health care professionals receive notification of deployment approximately six months prior to deployment. The PDS conference was designed, in part, to help improve the predictability of PROFIS and the timing of the notification. Once names have been locked into PDS, approximately one month after the PDS conference, changes to who is assigned to PROFIS positions require approval from MEDCOM (this approval process is called a reclama). Deploying units claim that the assignments still frequently change, and this creates problems for the units.

Health care professionals reported in our survey that they often received notification and orders for deployment late. Forty-five percent of PROFIS deployers received their official orders less than one month prior to departure, and 25 percent did not receive notification until one month or less from the time of departure (Figure 4.11). This late timing is associated with a high degree of dissatisfaction (Figure 4.12). Receiving orders late also hampers the ability of the PROFIS deployer to take care of personal business prior to deployment, such as breaking leases, putting household goods in storage, and tending to other personal affairs.

This late notice is partly due to approved reclamas. In some cases, reclamas are inevitable—a person develops a medical condition or gives notice that they are getting out of the U.S. Army. However, there are a large number of reclamas that do not fit those categories and are driven by the consultant or commander request (Figure 4.13). Additionally, our interviews suggest that not all deploying unit leaders understand the process for requesting PROFIS fillers, and delays in requesting the fillers are partly to blame for late notification.

Skills and Training

Skills and training are also issues that are important to both the health care professionals and the receiving units, although in different ways. The health care professionals want to be well trained for the position that they are getting ready to fill. This includes specific trauma, clinical, or surgical training that they might need to perform their duties. Receiving units want their PROFIS fillers to have the required clinical skills but, especially units other than CSHs, also want their health care professionals to have the appropriate soldier skills necessary to complete their tasks. For instance, receiving units mentioned that their PROFIS personnel did not all know how to wear their safety gear or enter and exit from a military vehicle correctly. Most personnel from the receiving units desired to have their PROFIS fillers arrive at least 30 days prior to deployment; however, the health care professionals often complained that there was not much to do during that time. Often, the receiving units were on block leave during much of that time, and the training that they needed to perform to get ready for deployment was not well organized. Health care professionals typically reported that the five-day training program

Figure 4.11
Reported Timing of Notification and Orders for PROFIS Personnel Prior to Deployment

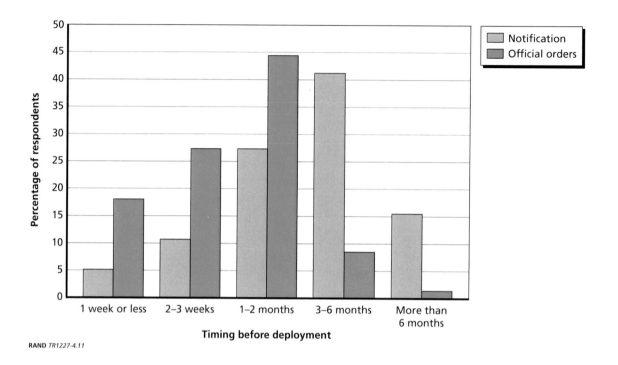

RAND TR1227-4.11

Figure 4.12
Satisfaction with Timing of Orders for Deployment

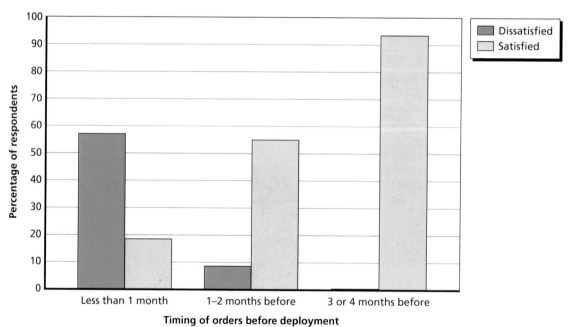

RAND TR1227-4.12

Figure 4.13
Total Number of Reclamas, by Year and Type of Request

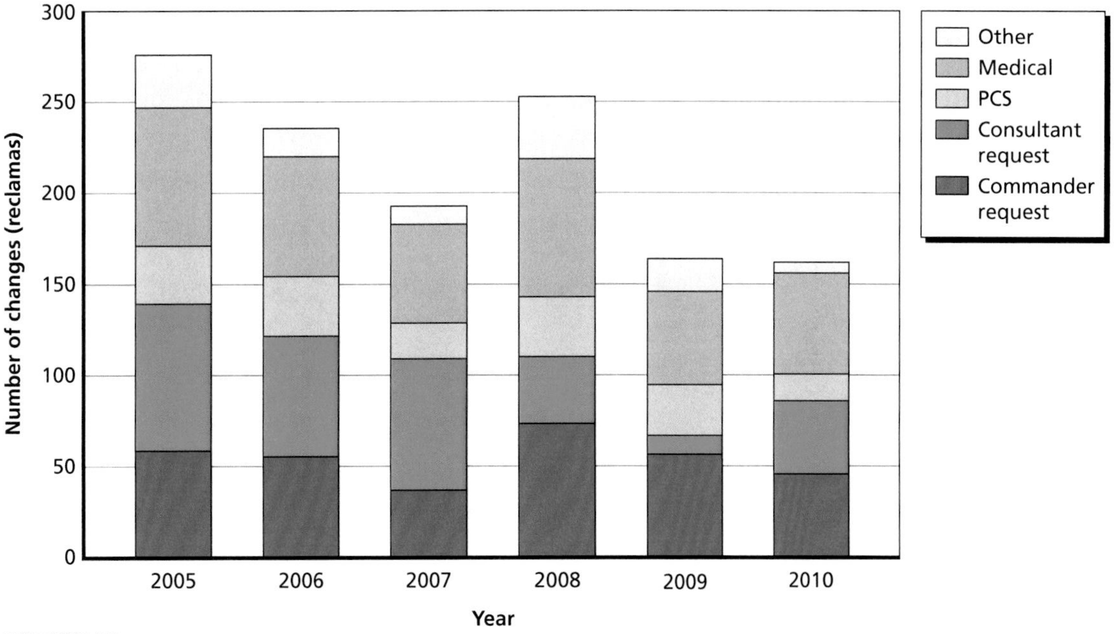

RAND TR1227-4.13

at the Continental U.S. Replacement Center at Fort Benning that is designed to prepare individuals meeting an already deployed unit was more streamlined and a better use of their time.

PROFIS fillers were more likely than organic health care professionals to report that participating in the culminating training exercise for their deploying unit is important (71–85 percent for PROFIS fillers, compared with 42–69 percent for organic health care professionals across corps). Across all the corps except the Veterinary Corps and Enlisted Corps, health care professionals reported that participating in soldier skills training is less important than the culminating training exercise. However, the culminating training exercise is not usually within the 30-day window prior to deployment, so this requires the PROFIS fillers to be released from their permanent duty station a separate time before deployment. PROFIS fillers also reported that the various clinical/surgical trauma courses that the U.S. Army offers are important, but some mentioned that they are only useful if PROFIS fillers complete the training with the same personnel they deploy with.

During deployment, some health care professionals, especially physicians (50 percent), reported that their clinical or surgical skills decreased. This could happen in two ways: either a skills mismatch between a physician and PROFIS position (e.g., a specialist being deployed in a battalion surgeon position where the specialist does not have the opportunity to practice his or her specialty) or low utilization (e.g., a surgeon being deployed to a forward surgical team or CSH that does not see a high patient load or does not see patients across the range of surgeries the surgeon normally performs). However, with the exception of the Medical Corps, more health care professionals reported that their clinical or surgical skills increased while deployed rather than decreased (Figure 4.14).[9] From our modeling, health care professionals who reported skills decreasing were more likely to view PROFIS as inequitable and were less likely to report intending to stay in the U.S. Army at the end of their ADSO. Within the Medical Corps, the procedure-intensive subspecialists[10] were most likely to report their clinical skills decreased (>80 percent). The vast majority of health care professionals across the corps reported that less than six months is the longest deployment that would not adversely affect their clinical skills (ranged from 68.2 percent of respondents in the Medical Specialist Corps to 90.4 percent of respondents in the Medical Corps who reported clinical skills degradation during their most recent deployment).

Not all deploying unit commanders and staff believe that physician skills decrease while deployed. They reported that some physicians can read journal articles while deployed, and one commander, whose battalion was on a larger base in Iraq, reported sending his battalion surgeon to the clinic and CSH on base during slow times to help her maintain skills. They did agree that the procedure-intensive subspecialists and surgeons could potentially lose some skills and dexterity during deployments. However, physicians reported during our interviews that, even when busy while deployed, they often were not seeing the same mix of cases that they would normally see at their permanent duty station. For instance, family physicians and obstetricians are not delivering babies while deployed, and surgeons are not performing laparo-

Figure 4.14
Impact of Deployment on Clinical and Surgical Skills

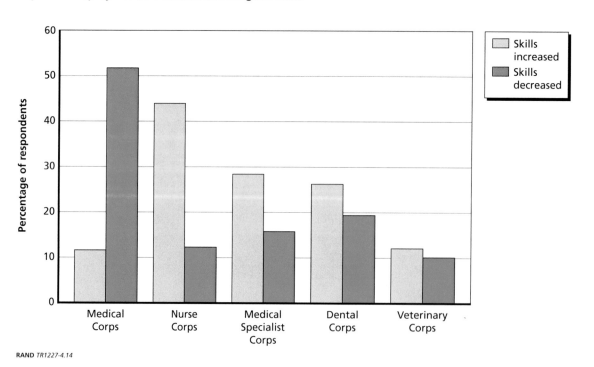

RAND TR1227-4.14

---

[9] The Enlisted Corps were not asked about their clinical and surgical skills.

[10] Procedure-intensive subspecialists for this analysis are cardiologists (60H), anesthesiologists (60N), gastroenterologists (60G), and dermatologists (60L).

scopic (fiber-optic) surgeries. The majority of survey respondents reported that six months was the longest they could be deployed without skills degradation (data not shown).

Once a deployment ends, the health care professionals must reintegrate into their assignment at their permanent duty station. Although there is a MEDCOM policy (Coley, 2009) on redeployment refresher training for physicians, our interviews indicated there is no standard way for this to occur. No set process exists for determining whether a health care professional's skills have degraded. The individual health care professional must notify his or her command of the skill decline. Because the returning health care professional's colleagues had often worked additional hours and cases while the PROFIS health care professional was deployed, some returning PROFIS fillers were hesitant to ask for lighter duty or extra help in regaining skills because of the extra burden that would place on their colleagues.

Survey respondents also reported on how deployment affects their leadership skills. Across all the corps, personnel reported that their leadership skills increased during deployment (Table 4.3). The percentage of respondents reporting that their leadership skills either increased or greatly increased ranged from about 57 percent for the Medical Corps to over 90 percent for the Enlisted Corps. These results are consistent with the information we heard during our interviews.

Impact on Military Treatment Facilities

MTF commanders and staff told us that PROFIS deployments have a substantial influence on their MTFs. They reported that deployments cause staffing vacancies that they frequently can not backfill, that deployments reduce access to care at the MTFs, with many cases being sent to the network, and that deployments might be having a negative effect on physician residency programs especially when there are not enough attending staff to maintain the volume of work required to train new physicians.

Our survey confirms that there is at least a perception of a negative effect on the MTFs. In most corps, at least 50 percent of the survey respondents reported that their workload increased when other personnel at their MTF were deployed, 30 to 65 percent reported that their work hours increased, and 15 to 50 percent reported a perception of decreased patient access (Figure 4.15). However, it should be noted that this is not a direct measure of patient access. Results from another, ongoing RAND study that is attempting to measure actual

Table 4.3
Impact of Deployment on Leadership Skills

Percentage Reported	Medical Corps	Nurse Corps	Medical Specialist Corps	Dental Corps	Veterinary Corps	Medical Service Corps	Enlisted Corps
Skills greatly increased	15.8	24.8	20.3	20.3	19.6	36.7	36.5
Skills increased	41.4	47.9	49.4	46.4	47.0	49.5	55.2
Skills neither increased nor decreased	27.5	22.4	24.2	28.3	29.3	10.9	7.3
Skills decreased	10.7	3.3	4.7	3.8	4.1	1.4	1.0
Skills greatly decreased	4.6	1.6	1.4	1.1	.	1.5	.

Figure 4.15
Impact of PROFIS Deployments on Military Treatment Facilities

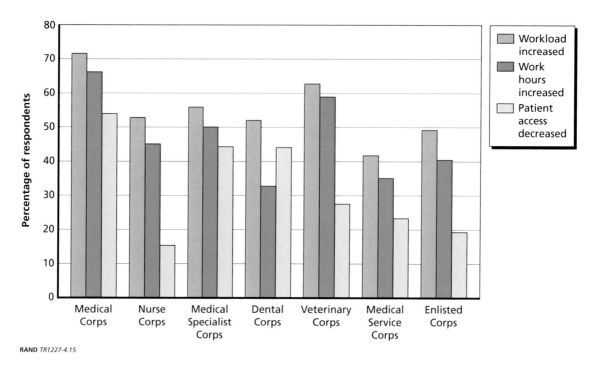

RAND TR1227-4.15

changes in TDA full-time-equivalent medical personnel and patient workloads at U.S. Army installations as a result of deployments suggest no significant overall access problems at the 14 installations examined.[11] This does not, however, preclude the existence of access-to-care issues for certain specialties or at other installations.

MTFs attempt to minimize the effect of PROFIS deployments by securing backfill for the health care professionals who have deployed. Early during OIF and OEF, Army Reserve units were called upon to provide backfill; however, individual reservists backfill for only 90 days. This is still the case in some corps, but in the Medical Corps and others, the reserve units have also been deploying frequently and do not have the ability to provide backfill to active units. So MTFs rely on civilian contracts for backfill. However, this process does not come close to filling all of the positions that are vacated due to deployments. Health care professionals who had personnel from their MTF deploy as PROFIS fillers reported that backfill ranged, depending on the corps, from 23 percent in the Medical Corps to a high of 71 percent in the Nurse Corps (Table 4.4). When backfill did occur, it frequently did not cover more than 50 percent of the time that the health care professional was deployed. However, when backfill did occur, generally the health care professionals were satisfied with the skills of the backfill provider and they were well integrated into the patient care team. Successful backfill mitigates the perceived impact of PROFIS deployments on the MTFs. Health care professionals who reported that their MTF received at least 50 percent backfill were less likely to report higher workload, more work hours, and decreased patient access (Table 4.4).

___

[11]   Adam Resnick, Mireille Jacobson, Spikanth Kadiyala, Nicole Eberhart, and Sue Hosek, unpublished RAND research, 2011.

Table 4.4
Rates, Impact, and Satisfaction of Backfill, by Corps

Percentage Reported	Medical Corps	Nurse Corps	Medical Specialist Corps	Dental Corps	Veterinary Corps	Medical Service Corps	Enlisted Corps
No backfill reported	63.7	28.8	47.9	77.3	72.8	46.4	51.3
Up to 50% backfill	22.7	37.4	26.0	*	*	26.0	28.2
Greater than 50% backfill	13.6	33.8	26.0	*	*	27.6	20.5
If >50% backfill reported							
Satisfied or very satisfied with skills of backfill provider	60.8	62.6	65.4	*	*	63.5	59.8
Backfill provider integrated very well or well into the patient care team	65.3	71.2	66.7	*	*	59.5	63.0
If >50% backfill							
Workload increased	60.0	48.4	47.4	*	*	32.2	36.1
Workhours increased	44.0	38.6	37.1	*	*	33.9	27.8
Reported patient access decreased	39.5	8.7	32.1	*	*	24.9	11.8
If <50% backfill							
Workload increased	69.2	52.6	54.8	*	*	40.9	49.4
Workhours increased	64.0	45.6	50.3	*	*	31.5	38.6
Reported patient access decreased	52.3	16.6	47.3	*	*	21.7	17.5

NOTE: * indicates a cell with fewer than 25 observations, which are not reported.

Retention

Views on retention varied among the senior leaders within AMEDD we interviewed. One person reported that retention goals have been exceeded in the past few years, but others said that not all residency positions are being filled, and they have heard anecdotal evidence that deployments are a major factor in the decision process for a health care professional to stay in or leave the Army. This, they report, is especially true for some of the AOCs with a high deployment burden, such as general surgeons, physician assistants, and nurse anesthetists, as well as AOCs filling battalion surgeon taskings.

Our survey results are consistent with the views reported to us during interviews about the link between deployment and retention. Medical Corps and Medical Specialist Corps health care professionals were more likely than those in other corps to report that they do not intend to remain in the Army at the end of their service obligation (46 and 38 percent respectively, $p < 0.001$, Figure 4.16). In addition, a higher proportion of health care professionals who felt that they had spent more time away from their PDS than expected reported that time away increased their desire to leave the Army, compared with those who did not report spending more time away than expected (Table 4.5). Also, one-quarter to one-third of health care profes-

Figure 4.16
Intentions of Health Care Professionals to Remain on Active Duty After Their Current Service Obligation Ends

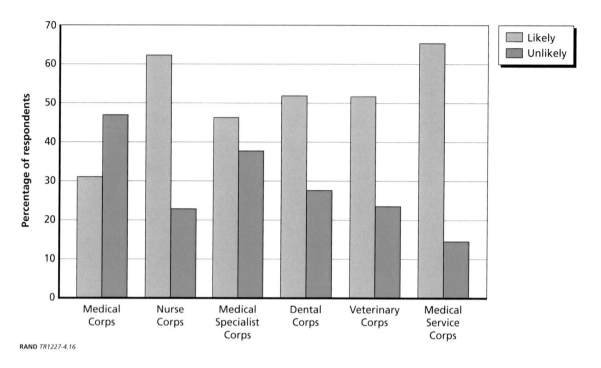

RAND *TR1227-4.16*

Table 4.5
Survey Respondent Retention Intentions

	Medical Corps	Nurse Corps	Medical Specialist Corps	Dental Corps	Veterinary Corps	Medical Service Corps	Enlisted Corps
How likely is it you will serve in military 20 years? (asked of everyone)							
Likely or very likely	40.9	65.6	61.5	44.9	52.8	67.8	70.7
Unlikely or very unlikely	38.8	19.8	21.8	38.0	18.3	17.1	19.0
Factors associated with retention intentions							
Time away from PDS somewhat or strongly increased desire to leave							
More time away than expected	71.5	36.1	76.8	*	*	32.6	*
Not more time away than expected	19.5	15.8	16.8	*	*	10.7	14.4
Spouse or significant other's view on remaining in Army							
Somewhat or strongly favors leaving	51.3	26.0	33.3	38.3	23.6	27.3	24.1
Somewhat or strongly favors remaining	25.9	42.0	41.9	37.7	37.3	49.9	47.1
Decreased desire to stay	16.3	15.3	16.4	21.7	47.5	18.1	30.6

NOTE: * indicates cells with fewer than 25 observations, which are not reported.

sionals in most corps reported that their spouse favored the health care professional leaving the Army, but over 50 percent of Medical Corps health care professional spouses are in favor of the respondent leaving the Army. Those whose spouses were dissatisfied or very dissatisfied with the support that was provided to their family while a health care professional was deployed thought their spouses were more likely to favor the health care professional leaving the Army than those whose spouses were satisfied or neither satisfied nor dissatisfied with the support provided to their family (Figure 4.17).

In multivariate analyses of the survey data, across most corps, some factors were consistently associated with our three measures of poor retention: (1) being unlikely or very unlikely to remain in the Army at the end of the ADSO, (2) being unlikely or very unlikely to stay in the Army for 20 years, and (3) reporting that time away from PDS increased desire to leave the military. Viewing PROFIS as inequitable (compared with viewing it as equitable or neutral) and reporting any skill loss while deployed (compared with reporting no impact on skill or skill increase) was statistically significantly associated with all three of the outcomes. In addition, for AMEDD personnel who had PROFIS personnel deploy from their MTF, reporting increased work hours due to that deployment was significantly associated with reduced retention intentions. These analyses controlled for tier and demographic and deployment characteristics (race, age, sex, marital status, dependents, rank, corps, and length of deployment).

While retention intentions are a useful indicator, they may or may not reflect actual behavior. We analyzed personnel data to understand what factors were associated with actually leaving the military. We examined the association between months deployed before the end of service obligation and retention in the Army, controlling for demographic factors, whether the

Figure 4.17
Effect of Satisfaction with Family Support on Spouses' Desire to Stay in or Leave the Army

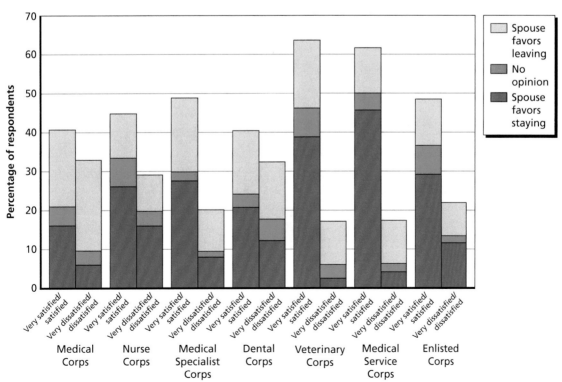

person's AOC was eligible for a bonus, and length of service when the person is first eligible to leave active duty. For enlisted soldiers, we examined the association between months deployed before their first ETS date and extending their service commitment after their ETS date. For officers, we examined the association between months deployed during their ADSO and time remaining on active duty after the completion of their ADSO.

The effect of deployment on retention is not the same for each corps. For the Nurse Corps and Medical Service Corps, more months spent deployed before the person's ADSO was associated with remaining on active duty longer after completion of their ADSO (Figure 4.18). For the Dental Corps, Veterinary Corps, and Medical Specialist Corps, deployment during ADSO was not associated with length of active duty service (data not shown). However, for the Medical Corps and Enlisted Corps, the relationship differs. For the Medical Corps, any deployment during their ADSO was significantly associated with leaving the military sooner after the ADSO (Figure 4.18). For the Enlisted Corps, we also found a significant negative relationship between number of months deployed and reenlistment (Figure 4.19 shows results by year that their first ETS date ended), with the effect of a deployment of at least seven months being associated with increasingly lower probability of remaining on active duty; we observe this effect until about 2006, after which the magnitude of the decrease remains approximately constant.[12] These data support the idea in the Medical Corps that deployment is a reason that physicians leave the Army. However, this is not the case for other officer corps, where deployment was reported in the interviews as often being seen as, or leading to, a leadership opportunity.

Summary of Key Observations

Key observations in the five areas we explored appear below.

Equity

- The corps with the highest percentage of deployed members are the Medical Specialist Corps, Enlisted Corps, and Medical Service Corps.
- The corps with the smallest percentage deployed are the Veterinary Corps and Dental Corps.
- The Medical Specialist Corps has deployed the most frequently (76 percent) and also has the most repeat deployers.
- In most AOCs, less than 10 percent of members have deployed two or more times.
- In some AOCs, at least 20 percent of members have deployed more than twice (with physician assistants and nurse anesthetists at over 50 percent, general surgeons at 46 percent, health care specialists at 28 percent, and health care administrators at 21 percent).
- Health care professionals are less likely to deploy if they are
  - female

---

[12] The Enlisted Corps analyses show a larger association between cumulative months of deployment prior to ETS date and leaving the Army than has been found in a previous RAND project that included all enlisted soldiers (Hosek and Martorell, 2009). Our analyses focus on the subset of enlisted soldiers that are part of AMEDD and covered a somewhat different time period than the other RAND study. The reason for the difference in these results is not entirely clear. It could be that the enlisted soldiers included in our analyses have better employment opportunities outside the Army compared with all enlisted personnel, or the difference could be due to slight variations in model specification or other unidentified reasons.

Figure 4.18
Survival Curves Describing Months Deployed Prior to End of ADSO and Percentage Staying in the Army After ADSO for Officers

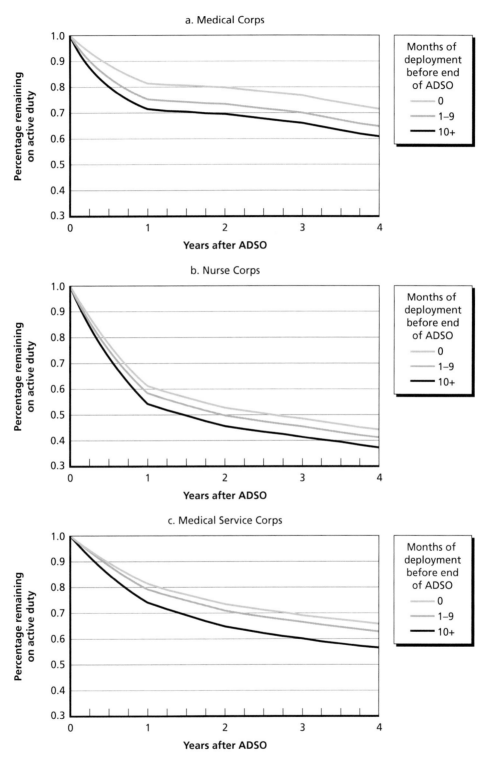

Figure 4.19
Estimated Effects of Cumulative Months of Deployment on the Percentage of Enlisted Corps Choosing to Reenlist at the First Reenlistment Decision, Over Time

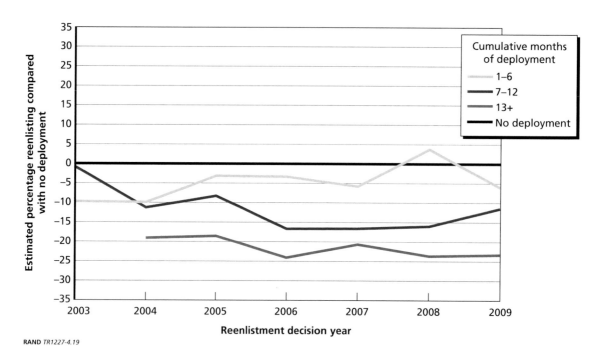

RAND *TR1227-4.19*

- black and in the Nurse Corps, Medical Service Corps, or Enlisted Corps; or Hispanic in the Nurse Corps
  - O-5 or above and in the Nurse Corps, Medical Specialist Corps, or Dental Corps.
- Health care professionals are more likely to deploy if they
  - are a senior enlisted personnel (E-5 and above).
- Most survey respondents regarded PROFIS as equitable or said they do not know whether it is.
- More than one-third of the Medical Corps said that PROFIS is inequitable.
- Those in battalion surgeon positions tend to deploy longer than those in other Medical Corps positions and were more likely to see PROFIS as inequitable.

Predictability

- PROFIS does not currently achieve its goal of establishing predictability among health care professionals and receiving units:
  - 45 percent of the PROFIS deployers receive their orders one month or less from their deployment date.
  - Some late notifications result from reclamas or failure on the part of the deploying unit to request PROFIS soon enough.

Skills and Training

- Some personnel, especially physicians, reported skill degradation.
- There is no systematic process for determining whether skills have degraded.
- More than 60 percent in all corps reported that their *leadership* skills increased.

Impact on Military Treatment Facilities

- Health care professionals at MTFs reported significant effects on MTFs from PROFIS deployments:
    - many vacated positions not backfilled
    - higher workload and increased work hours
    - perception of reduced access to care
    - backfills that do not cover the full period of absence.

Retention

- The following correlated with poor retention intentions:
    - seeing PROFIS as inequitable
    - reporting skills degradation while deployed
    - reporting increased work hours due to others being deployed from the MTF.
- This effect of deployment on retention intentions varies by corps:
    - For the Nurse Corps, Medical Service Corps, and Medical Specialist Corps, more months spent deployed before ADSO was associated with remaining on active duty after ADSO.
    - For the Medical Corps, any deployment was associated with leaving the military sooner after ADSO.

In the next chapter, we describe potential modifications to PROFIS that could potentially address the issues identified in this chapter. We also describe our qualitative assessment of how the potential modifications would affect relevant stakeholders.

CHAPTER FIVE

Potential Modifications to PROFIS

In this chapter, we describe potential modifications to PROFIS that could address some of the issues raised in Chapter Four. Generally, PROFIS works as designed, allowing medical personnel to work in fixed facilities primarily and then supplement deploying units as necessary. We do not think that abandoning PROFIS is necessary, but these modifications could improve the system from a variety of stakeholder viewpoints. The modifications would need to work under the current deployment circumstances, under conditions when PROFIS fillers are not deploying frequently, and under the conditions to support a very large-scale, short-notice deployment.

We did not formally analyze or model these modifications. We conducted qualitative assessments to assess how they might affect different stakeholders. However, we recommend more formal assessments before any modification is implemented. These modifications were suggested by individuals we interviewed, were written about in informal papers, are practiced by our allies, or were developed by the RAND team.

We summarized the issues that were raised regarding PROFIS into five categories (see Table 4.1): equity, predictability, skills and training, impact on the MTFs, and retention. Many of the modifications address multiple issues or concerns. As a result, we categorized modifications differently (Table 5.1), assessing whether they

1. increase supply of providers available for deployment
2. change the battalion surgeon position
3. improve predictability
4. improve backfill
5. reduce skills degradation
6. improve other equity issues.

We then assessed qualitatively how each modification might affect different stakeholders and which of the five issues they address. For health care professionals, we focused on the impact a change would have on equity; deployment issues, such as skills match and degradation; and retention. For the MTFs, we considered how leadership and management of the facilities might view the change: How would these changes affect the staffing at their facilities, would it be easier or harder to fill PROFIS positions they are assigned, etc. For the regional medical commands, we considered how the changes would likely affect how they manage their specific PROFIS requirements. From the AMEDD perspective, we considered how changes would affect the personnel who are running and managing PROFIS as well as such considerations as accession of health care professionals. For the receiving units, we considered the effect of the changes on the leadership and soldiers of those units.

Table 5.1
Potential Modifications to PROFIS and Their Qualitative Impacts

Category	Potential Modification	Issues Affected
Increase supply of health care professionals available for deployment	Limit the number of consecutive assignments to nondeployable positions (e.g., Office of the Surgeon General, DCCS, DCN).	Equity; impact on MTFs, retention
	Limit the number of personnel with nondeployable profiles assigned to deployable positions. (Assign personnel with nondeployable profiles to "fenced positions" or other nondeployable positions.)	Equity; impact on MTFs; retention
	Offer better rewards for deployment (e.g., prioritize for first choice on next permanent change of station).	Equity; retention
	Delay fellowships. (Require certain number of years of practice in general specialty before allowing subspecialization.)	Equity; skills and training; impact on MTFs; retention
	Shift the requirements for number of personnel in each AOC to increase personnel in AOCs in higher demand for deployment (e.g., increase supply of physician assistants or general surgeons).	Equity; skills and training; impact on MTFs; retention
	Offer long-term civilian contracts for Army-trained subspecialists (all corps).	Equity; skills and training; impact on MTFs; retention
	Deploy civilian volunteers to CSHs (similar to approach of some other countries).	Equity; skills and training; impact on MTFs; retention
Change the battalion surgeon position	Provide short-term "retraining" before deployment (for subspecialists and nonpracticing MDs) (focusing on sick call, trauma, deployed medicine).	Skills and training
	Implement 6-month deployments for all PROFIS battalion surgeons.	Equity; impact on MTFs; retention
	Direct Army-trained interns to practice as general medical officers for 1–2 years before finishing residency (in either MTF or FORSCOM positions).	Equity; predictability; skills and training; impact on MTFs; retention
	Fill all battalion surgeon PROFIS positions with physician assistants and nurse practitioners (depending on substitutability). (This would require increase in physician assistant/nurse practitioner manning.)	Equity; skills and training; impact on MTFs; retention
	Use a borrowed military manpower system for battalion surgeons. (Providers assigned permanently to battalion surgeon positions, but must work part-time at local MTF.)	Equity; skills and training; impact on MTFs; retention
Improve predictability	Improve timeliness of cutting of orders for PROFIS personnel.	Predictability
	Move PDS conference timing 1 month earlier each year or do it in person more frequently (e.g., 2 in person per year and 1 by email). (This would better match deployment cycle.)	Predictability
	Offer long-term PROFIS assignments (PROFIS positions assigned for 3–4 years regardless of whether personnel change duty stations).	Predictability
	Follow the Army ARFORGEN cycle for PROFIS positions and personnel. (Do not assign PROFIS personnel to units during reset period of ARFORGEN.)	Equity; predictability; retention
	Use a borrowed military manpower system for all PROFIS positions. (Providers assigned permanently to deploying units, but must work part-time at local MTF.)	Equity; predictability; retention

Table 5.1—Continued

Category	Potential Modification	Issues Affected
Reduce impact of deployment on MTFs	Increase civilian staff at MTFs.	Impact on MTFs
	Use national backfill contract for regional medical commands/MTFs.	Impact on MTFs
Reduce skills degradation	Have no deployment in year following residency (any kind of major training). (This would allow skills to solidify before deployments.)	Equity; skills and training; impact on MTFs; retention
	Provide more formal reassessment of staff skills upon redeployment.	Skills and training; impact on MTFs; retention
Improve other equity issues	Eliminate 90-day post-stabilization redeployment period for 62B and behavioral health specialties.	Equity; impact on MTFs; retention
	Switch all officer AOCs to Tier I and manage centrally.	Equity; predictability

We present this assessment as simple categories of effect: improves, neutral, worsens, or a combination. In some cases, we assess the change as both "improves" and "worsens." This can mean that the change might improve the situation for some individuals within a group of stakeholders (e.g., a specific group of AOCs) but worsen it for others; or it can mean that there are multiple effects, and some would be an improvement and some would make things worse. We did not assess how many people within a category would be affected by the change. We also focused on primary effects, understanding that some changes might have downstream impacts that affect more categories. The rest of this chapter describes these modifications and their potential effect in more detail.

Increase the Supply of Providers Available for Deployment

Some of the issues surrounding equity—who deploys and how often they are deployed—can be addressed by increasing the supply of providers available for deployment (Table 5.2). For our analysis, we assume that the total strength of AMEDD will not change, so increasing the supply of personnel in a specific AOC/MOS would generally require reducing the supply of health care professionals in other AOCs. Some of the potential modifications to increase supply are minor, while others would require larger changes in AMEDD policies and procedures.

Limit Consecutive Assignments in Nondeployable Positions

In some corps, personnel in specific positions are treated as nondeployable; for instance, we were informed that many hospitals treat their DCCSs and DCNs as not available for deployment. Although we do not have quantitative data to support this, we heard in our interviews and from written comments in the survey that some personnel take advantage of this by moving from one nondeployable position to another. A policy that limits the number of consecutive assignments health care professionals can serve in nondeployable positions would increase the equity of deployments by increasing the number of people in the deployment pool. It is not clear how many positions are deemed nondeployable by commands, so this might have more of an impact on perceptions of equity than actual deployments for individual health care professionals. This could be positive for the MTFs if perceptions of equity improved, since that could improve working conditions. Also, the burden of deployment would be spread across

Table 5.2
Assessment of Potential Modifications to Increase the Supply of Health Care Professionals Available for Deployment

Potential Modification	Health Care Professional	MTF	Regional Medical Command	AMEDD Leadership	Receiving Unit
Limit consecutive assignments in nondeployable positions (e.g., Office of the Surgeon General, DCCS, DCN).	Improves for some health care professionals and worsens for others	Improves and worsens	Improves	Improves	Neutral
Reduce nondeployable profiles in deployable positions. (Assign personnel with nondeployable profiles to "fenced positions" or other nondeployable positions.)	Improves for some health care professionals and worsens for others	Improves and worsens	Improves	Improves	Neutral
Improve rewards for deployment (e.g., prioritize for first choice on next permanent change of station).	Improves	Neutral	Neutral	Neutral	Neutral
Delay fellowships (require X years practice in general specialty before allowing subspecialization).	Worsens	Improves and worsens	Improves	Improves and worsens	Improves
Shift requirements to increase AOCs in demand (e.g., increase supply of physician assistants or general surgeons).	Improves for some health care professionals and worsens for others	Worsens	Improves	Improves and worsens	Neutral
Offer long-term civilian contracts for Army-trained subspecialists (all corps; pediatric oncologists, etc.).	Improves	Improves	Improves	Neutral	Improves
Deploy civilians to CSHs. (This is similar to approach of some other countries.)	Improves for some health care professionals and slightly worsens for others	Improves	Improves and worsens	Improves and worsens	Worsens

more people, potentially, so MTF and regional medical command leadership would have more options in terms of people who have not recently deployed to send on deployment. This could have a negative effect on the specific individuals who are being asked to move out of nondeployable positions, and it could have a negative impact on the MTFs that may value specific individuals in these leadership positions.

Reduce Nondeployable Profiles in Deployable Positions

Reducing the number of personnel with nondeployable profiles who are in deployable positions is another potential modification. There are a number of personnel who may be highly valued in the Army, but are unable to deploy for a medical reason. There are also positions, either by policy or by practice, that are not used to fill PROFIS positions. These include the examples above as well as informal positions that regional medical commands have "fenced." Some consultants and regional medical command commanders will not deploy a health care professional from a medical facility if that person is one of only one or two health care professionals in that specialty in the facility and if the civilian network in the area is weak. For instance, the Western Regional Medical Command tries not to deploy physicians from Fort Wainwright in Alaska. For AOCs that are in high demand for deployment, the Army could assign personnel with permanent profiles (e.g., they can never deploy) to the positions that are nondeployable by policy or by practice. By pairing nondeployable health care professionals with nondeployable positions, the total number of people available to deploy would increase. This would generally be positive for individual health care professionals, except perhaps for those that are sent to a location they view as undesirable. Similarly MTFs would have more personnel available for deployment, but might lose some senior personnel with permanent profiles who are transferred to other locations. Another possibility would be to utilize nondeployable health care professionals as backfill for personnel who are deployed from locations that are currently "fenced."

Improve Rewards for Deployment

Another potential modification is to provide better rewards for deployments. This could be in terms of deployers getting priority consideration for their first choice for their next duty station, or getting priority for their first choice for additional education or school. A potential negative effect of this is that it might increase the likelihood that nondeployers leave the Army if they are not getting their choice of duty station or school.

Delay Fellowships

In corps that have subspecialty training, one option for increasing the supply of personnel available to deploy is to delay subspecialty fellowship training. This would not increase the total supply of health care professionals, but it would increase the early career supply of the more generalist types (e.g., general surgeon, internal medicine physicians, general dentists, medical-surgical nurses). This could affect health care professionals negatively, in that they will not be able to subspecialize as early in their career, which could reduce retention or could even reduce accession, if physicians in training choose not to join the Army because it would take them longer to become specialty trained than it would in another service or as a civilian. It could also potentially reduce the supply of specialists for the Army medical centers and teaching facilities. These effects would be of concern to AMEDD leadership, and could have a negative impact on MTFs if there are fewer subspecialists to fill positions in medical centers.

The next three modifications would require substantial shifts in doctrine and manning, but all have greater potential to reduce the deployment inequities.

Shift Requirements to Increase AOCs in Demand

Because there is a wide range of deployment rates between different AOCs (see Figure 4.2), the Army could increase the number of personnel in the AOCs in high demand and decrease the number of personnel in AOCs in low demand. For instance, AMEDD could reduce the number of pathologists and radiologists in the Army. These specialties are not in high demand in the deployed environment, although they are important in the medical centers. Those spots could then be shifted to general surgeons or internists or other AOCs with a higher deployment frequency. Similar shifts could occur in other corps.

Two potential negative effects were voiced by medical corps leadership. First, since residency programs need subspecialists to help with physician training, this could have an adverse effect on residency program staffing. Second, reducing the specialties not in demand for deployment could reduce the ability to provide comprehensive care in MTFs. This modification would likely have to occur in conjunction with hiring more civilian health care professionals at MTFs in the specialties that are being reduced in the Army to alleviate these concerns.

One of the other concerns with this modification is that it could reduce the ability of the AMEDD to recruit health care professionals. AMEDD might not be able to fill its authorizations if young health care professionals, especially physicians, have more limited choice of specialty in which they can train, or if the difficulty of being selected for training in certain specialties is increased. Another issue that would have to be assessed is whether there is sufficient demand in the nondeployed settings to appropriately utilize the increased supply of professionals in high demand for deployment AOCs. This increase could improve situations at MTFs, since there would be more health care professionals available for deployment in high-demand positions, or it could create challenges if there is not enough volume at the MTFs for the extra health care professionals to be productive and maintain their skills.

Offer Long-Term Civilian Contracts

A related modification to the one above is to change how the Army employs certain subspecialists. There seems to be a need and desire to have subspecialists practicing in MTFs, but the demand for many of these specialties in deployed settings is low. The AMEDD could continue to train subspecialists, but, instead of serving only on active duty after training, those specialists could serve at least part of their ADSO through long-term civilian contracts providing care at MTFs. This would allow the Army to continue to recruit top health care professionals with an interest in specialty training, it would allow the Army to utilize health care professionals' skills where they are in demand (in the MTFs), and it would allow AMEDD leadership to increase the number of positions that could be filled by health care professionals in high-demand AOCs. This modification provides added benefit because the receiving units would not be getting subspecialists filling positions that should be filled by more generalists, thereby improving the skills match between task and health care professional.

Deploy Civilians to Combat Support Hospitals

A final modification to increase the supply of health care professionals available for deployment is to utilize civilians in some deployed positions. This would be similar to what Canada and the Netherlands do, in part, to staff their deployed hospitals. It would likely only work in specific situations, mostly CSHs. The length of deployments might need to be shorter—the civilians deploying in Canada go for four weeks. It could increase costs, because the Army would likely have to pay substantial bonuses to encourage civilians to deploy to combat zones and would have to pay a competitive salary, which might be higher in the private sector. This might require civilians to go through a formal short course in military medicine and general military training prior to deployment.

Make Changes to the Battalion Surgeon Position

As described in Chapter Four, the battalion surgeon position is a special case that creates substantial issues. Here we describe five potential changes to the battalion surgeon position that may improve numerous aspects of the position (Table 5.3). These range from the type of train-

Table 5.3
Assessment of Potential Modifications That Change the Battalion Surgeon Position

Potential Modification	Health Care Professional	MTF	Regional Medical Command	AMEDD Leadership	Receiving Unit
Create a battalion surgeon training module (for subspecialists and nonpracticing MDs) emphasizing sick call, trauma, deployed medicine.	Improves	Worsens	Neutral	Neutral	Improves
Shorten battalion surgeon deployment length.	Improves	Improves	Improves	Improves	Worsens
Have interns practice as general medical officers prior to completing residency (in either MTF or FORSCOM positions).	Worsens	Worsens	Worsens	Worsens	Worsens
Use physician extenders as battalion surgeons. (This would require increase in physician assistant manning and altering substitutability for nurse practitioners.)	Improves	Improves	Improves	Improves	Improves
Use a borrowed military manpower system for battalion surgeons. (Providers assigned permanently to battalion surgeon positions, but must work part time at local MTF.)	Worsens	Worsens	Neutral	Worsens	Improves

ing battalion surgeons receive, to the length of their deployments, to what types of health care professionals fill the battalion surgeon position.

Create a Battalion Surgeon Training Module

Currently, primary care physicians and many subspecialists can deploy as battalion surgeons (see Figure 4.6). However, the role of the battalion surgeon does not generally include subspecialty care delivery. Battalion surgeons are called on to perform a variety of duties, including manning the battalion aid station, supervising physician assistants and medics, and advising battalion leadership on medical issues. Most of the medical care is limited to light trauma and sick call type issues. In our survey, physicians who deployed as battalion surgeons were more likely to report not being well prepared for their clinical duties while deployed. Our first potential modification is to develop a short training course on battalion surgeon duties. This would be offered to subspecialists and nonpracticing medical doctors (MDs) (research physicians who are not typically seeing patients) to allow them to refresh their sick call and trauma treatment skills. This might be considered worse for the MTFs, since they would potentially lose these physicians for a longer period of time due to the training. Physicians might see this as an improvement if they perceived it as useful and not too long.

Shorten Battalion Surgeon Deployment Length

Physicians deployed as battalion surgeons have been required to stay with their deployed unit for 12 months as well as up to 90 days post-deployment during a stabilization period. However, the Army moved to a standard 9-month deployment schedule for many units starting April 2012. Twelve-month deployments have led to reported skills degradation, even among generalists if they are not seeing the range of cases they normally see in the clinic or MTF.

Battalion surgeons were able to apply for an exception to policy to split their deployment after 6 months with another physician if they were experiencing skill degradation or had another reason to request it. We suggest investigating the feasibility of limiting deployments for all battalion surgeons to no more than six months. If a physician wants to stay for longer, he or she can request an extension. This also is more closely aligned with how other services deploy physicians. This change will be perceived as worse for the receiving units, which typically like to have their battalion surgeon stay with them for the duration of their deployment. ALARACT 013/2012, which affected deployments as of February 1, 2012, reduced PROFIS deployments to 270 days, and Medical Corps and Dental Corps officers now deploy for 135 days if assigned to PROFIS positions in medical brigades or units echelon above brigade.

Have Interns Practice as General Medical Officers Prior to Completing Residency

The Army, Air Force, and Navy all used to utilize general medical officers, physicians who had completed a one-year clinical internship but not residency training programs, in many medical positions. These general medical officers provided general care to patients and input to military leadership on medical issues. Over time, the military services have largely phased out the general medical officer positions. However, one option for the battalion surgeon position is to reintroduce the general medical officer practice. All, or a large subset, of Army-trained physicians could be asked to practice for one to two years as a battalion surgeon prior to completing residency training in their chosen specialty. These physicians would be assigned to organic positions after completing their internship year and would practice for one to two years as general medical officers, seeing patients in the troop clinics and sick call, etc. While this would reduce the number of subspecialists being assigned to these positions during deployment, it would also assign a physician with much less training than the current system does. In addition, non–primary care physicians (e.g., surgeons, OB/GYNs, dermatologists) would have completed an intern year that might not include much training in the type of medicine that they would be required to perform as a general medical officer. This could potentially affect the quality of care that is delivered by battalion surgeons. In our estimation, this would actually be a worse system for all, or almost all, of the stakeholders. Physicians would not want to delay residency training. If they had to, then more could possibly choose to extend as a general medical officer and leave the military as soon as their service obligation is completed. Receiving units would receive physicians who have completed fewer years of training and have less experience treating patients.

Use Physician Extenders as Battalion Surgeons

The current system utilizes a physician assistant as the battalion surgeon while the unit is in garrison. Once the unit receives its PROFIS personnel for deployment, a PROFIS physician fills the battalion surgeon position. However, the physician assistant is possibly as well as or better prepared than the physician for the role of a battalion surgeon in terms of the type of care that is required and the fit with the receiving unit. One potential modification is to switch the battalion surgeon position to a senior physician assistant position (Malish, 2009). In this case, a battalion would have one physician assistant who is assigned organically and a second physician assistant who is assigned by PROFIS.

This modification has multiple potentially positive outcomes. The physician assistants have more specific training in sick call and trauma care than many physician specialties who fill the battalion surgeon positions, they have more experience working with FORSCOM and other TOE units, and they often have prior Army experience and understand Army culture better than some of the PROFIS physicians. In fact, some of the physicians we interviewed who had filled battalion surgeon roles reported that their physician assistants were better trained in battlefield medicine than they were. Furthermore, a recent study that surveyed 13 physician assistants and 13 physicians deployed in combat positions in 2010 found that physician assistants rated physician assistants as better prepared for core battalion medical mission than physicians, while physicians viewed physician assistants and physicians as equally prepared (Malish et al., 2011). In the civilian literature, researchers have demonstrated that nurse practitioners and physician assistants provide similar quality of care to physicians (Sox, 1979; Hooker and Berlin, 2002; Roy et al., 2008). However, physician assistants are already the most deployed AOC within AMEDD, so this would require a significant increase in the number of physician assistants in the Army. Keeping AMEDD manning constant, this would require shifting requirements from other corps to the Medical Specialist Corps. However, it might be possible to utilize more physician assistants throughout MEDCOM, in MTFs and other clinics to perform primary care. That is a growing trend in civilian health care (Hooker and Berlin, 2002; Druss et al., 2003) that the Army might choose to copy. This is also a potential cost-saving strategy, since training physician assistants is likely less expensive than training physicians.

Utilizing physician assistants as battalion surgeons deployed might also require a change in how the physician assistants are supervised while deployed. The supervision of physician assistants by physicians in the Army falls under AR 40-68 as well as the laws of the individual state in which the physician assistant is practicing (AR 40-68, 2009). AR 40-68 (p. 41) states that

> the supervising physician must, when needed, prescribe standards of good medical practice. The supervisor must be available for consultation in person, telephonically, by radio, or by any other means that allows person-to-person exchange of information.

Currently, the PROFIS battalion surgeon provides that supervision. With this proposed change, the battalion surgeons would need to be supervised by another physician, potentially the brigade surgeon. However, if this supervisory responsibility increases the brigade surgeon's workload substantially, then the Army could add a PROFIS-assigned assistant brigade surgeon, as a PROFIS position. As there are often 5–6 battalions in each brigade, this would still significantly reduce the number of PROFIS physician positions while still, potentially, providing health care professionals who are a better fit for the receiving units.

In addition to considering physician assistants for battalion surgeon positions, the AMEDD could consider using family nurse practitioners in these positions. They would likely require more trauma care training and would also require an increase in manning. However, the physician supervision requirements are not as stringent as those for physician assistants.

Use Borrowed Military Manpower for Battalion Surgeons

Another potential change to the battalion surgeon position would be to change it to an organic position, but require the individuals assigned as battalion surgeons to work a substantial part of their time in garrison at an MTF (the Borrowed Military Manpower model). This would mitigate the issues that the receiving units have expressed about PROFIS providers, for example, concerns about soldier skills training and suboptimal integration with the unit. This approach, however, would likely be seen as a much worse situation by the health care professionals themselves, since they could have substantially less time in the clinic and could experience skills degradation if the unit did not release them to the MTF for an adequate amount of time or they were not fully utilized at the MTF. Similarly, this would be worse for MTFs, which would have fewer physician resources. Borrowed military manpower would work best if a policy was agreed upon by AMEDD and FORSCOM leadership and was set for the minimum amount of time that health care professionals were required to spend in an MTF and the type of clinic they provide that care in (e.g., clinics seeing families and retirees, not just in troop-only clinics). However, the health care professionals would be subject to the authority of the battalion commander, who might well ignore the opportunity cost—negative effects for the MTF and the health care professional's skills retention—in deciding what duties the commander wanted the health care professional to perform.

Improve Predictability of PROFIS

Many of the issues described in Chapter Four regarding PROFIS and how it is implemented involve the predictability of the system. Figures 4.9 and 4.10 highlight the importance of notification and receiving orders on satisfaction with PROFIS. And a common complaint from receiving units is that the health care professionals assigned to their PROFIS requirements changed frequently, and often at the last minute. We describe five modifications that could potentially improve some of the predictability issues (Table 5.4).

Improve Timeliness of Orders

One simple modification is to improve the timeliness of the receipt of orders for PROFIS deployments by health care professionals. From our interviews, it appears that MTFs and regional medical commands have little control over the actual cutting of orders, but that delays in cutting orders play a large role in PROFIS deployers not receiving orders in a timely manner. There is sometimes a substantial delay between when health care professionals receive verbal or

Table 5.4
Assessment of Potential Modifications to Improve the Predictability of PROFIS

Potential Modification	Health Care Professional	MTF	Regional Medical Command	AMEDD Leadership	Receiving Unit
Improve timeliness of orders for PROFIS personnel.	Improves	Improves	Improves	Improves	Improves
Change the frequency and/or timing of the PDS Conference (to better match deployment cycle).	Neutral/improves	Improves	Improves	Improves	Improves
Implement long-term PROFIS assignments (PROFIS positions assigned for 3–4 years regardless of if personnel permanent change of station).	Improves	Improves	Improves/worsens	Worsens	Improves
Implement ARFORGEN Cycle for PROFIS positions (remove names during reset).	Improves	Improves	Improves	Improves	Improves
Use a borrowed military manpower system for all PROFIS positions. (Providers assigned permanently to deploying units, but must work part-time at local MTF.)	Worsens	Worsens	Worsens	Worsens	Improves

email notification of deployment and when they receive their written orders. Personnel cannot take care of organizing their personal lives, including placing household goods into storage and addressing housing issues, until they have written orders. Interviews with individuals in human resources operations branch and MEDCOM Current Operations indicated that it is MEDCOM policy that everyone has their orders 30 days before they join their unit. Health care professionals, in theory, can delay their deployments until the 30 days have passed, but many may not be comfortable taking advantage of this option and joining their unit in theater 2–3 weeks after it deployed. One MTF told us that it has the capability to cut the orders in house, and it reported no delay in personnel receiving orders. Improving the timeliness of written orders would have the most impact on individual providers, but would also likely improve the situation for all stakeholders. We did not explore whether this would have an impact on other stakeholders, not identified here, including the commands/offices that actually write and deliver the orders.

Change the Frequency and/or Timing of PDS Conference

Another potential change to improving notification is to change the frequency or timing of the annual PDS conference. Because units overlap for a few weeks in theater, the cycle of deployments changes every year, with deployments happening on average a month earlier (Goymerak, 2007). The PDS conference was designed to identify which units were preparing to deploy eight or nine months in the future. However, since the timing of the PDS conference does not change, the units that are getting filled with PROFIS at the conference are potentially deploying closer to the PDS conference, leaving less notification time. Approximately six months after the PDS conference, the PDS conference attendees manage deployment assignments for off-cycle deployments over email (a virtual PDS conference), but it is not clear how well unit deployments are managed and how far in advance PROFIS personnel are being assigned to the units.

The two other potential modifications to the predictability of PROFIS involve how personnel are assigned to PROFIS positions. Currently, health care professionals are assigned based on the tier of the PROFIS position (I, II, III). Tier I positions are assigned by the consultant to the Army Surgeon General for that AOC. These are basically managed at the MEDCOM level. Tier II and III positions are distributed to the regional medical commands, which fill the positions or distribute them to the MTFs to fill. For Tier II and III, if a person is assigned to a PROFIS position and moves to a new duty station, then a new person needs to be assigned by the regional medical command/MTF to that PROFIS position.

Implement Long-Term PROFIS Assignments

An alternative way to manage PROFIS would be to assign personnel to PROFIS positions for approximately three-year periods—mirroring the 1:2 deployment-to-at-home ratio that ARFORGEN is trying to maintain. This would improve predictability from both the health care professional standpoint and the receiving unit standpoint. To work, however, positions that are typically split into two six-month deployments would need to have two people assigned to them.[1] This might be advantageous, because both individuals who would be deploying would

---

[1]   With the recent change in the Army to nine-month deployments, it is not clear whether some PROFIS positions will still be split between two deployers (two 4.5-month deployments) or all health care professionals will now complete full nine-month deployments.

potentially be available to go to training exercises with the unit. One negative aspect of this change is that it complicates the assignment of personnel to MTFs. AMEDD would need to consider a health care professional's PROFIS assignment when making permanent duty assignment decisions, to avoid too many people at one MTF being assigned to PROFIS positions in the same unit. This modification might also add work for the MTFs and regional medical commands, which would now have to track their personnel as they enter the region, making sure they know what PROFIS assignments they have.

Implement ARFORGEN Cycle for PROFIS Positions

Finally, a similar change would be to try to more closely follow the Army Force Generation (ARFORGEN) cycle in MEDCOM. ARFORGEN consists of three phases to prepare a unit for deployment: reset/train, ready, and available. Upon returning from a deployment, a unit enters the reset/train phase. Then the unit enters the ready phase, during which time it conducts mission training and preparation. Finally, the unit enters the available phase, where it is available to conduct deployment missions. During the reset period of ARFORGEN, units do not have a manning goal. At the start of the train/ready period, the manning goal is 80 percent but increases to >90 percent during that time (Casey, 2010). Finally, during the available period, the manning goal is 100–105 percent.

Currently, PROFIS positions are always "filled" for units, meaning they always have a name assigned to a PROFIS position. However, when a unit is actually identified to deploy, its PROFIS positions are moved into PDS and many, if not all, of the names assigned to the PROFIS positions are removed, and new personnel are assigned to these positions. This creates a lot of turmoil from the perspective of the receiving unit. During our interviews, we learned that it is common for the consultants and regional medical commands to assign, to PROFIS positions, personnel whom they know will not be able to deploy with those units due to profiles, protected positions, upcoming change of duty station, retirement, etc. They know those names will be removed and they can then assign a new person to the position when the unit is getting ready to deploy.

Not assigning PROFIS personnel during the reset period and for the initial part of the training period could reduce the number of name changes that occur once a unit is placed into PDS. It would also give health care professionals more predictability in terms of their deployments. And it might allow them to train more effectively with their units. Potentially, similar to the last modification, if the Army continues to split nine-month deployments, as they do 12-month deployments for some positions, two people could be assigned to each PROFIS position that is known to be a split-deployment position, again allowing both personnel to do some training with the unit. This would potentially improve the system for receiving units, if it reduces the frequency of names being changed in their PROFIS positions.

Use Borrowed Military Manpower for All Health Care Personnel

Earlier in this chapter, we described borrowed military manpower for the battalion surgeon position. Borrowed military manpower could also be implemented for all health care providers; this would assign providers permanently to deployable units and require them to work most of their time in garrison at the MTF or base clinic. As with borrowed military manpower for battalion surgeon positions, this would mitigate the issues that the receiving units have expressed about PROFIS providers, for example, concerns about the training on basic soldier skills, such as handling weapons and traveling in military transport vehicles, and suboptimal integration with the unit, and would reduce uncertainty about when health care professionals were going to be deployed. There are a number of downsides to this approach. Health care professionals' permanent assignments would be with their deploying unit. This may or may not be where their clinical skills are needed in the MTF system, which could result in further mismatches between health care professionals' clinical skills and their assignments, potentially leading to skills degradation. Health care professionals would also likely spend less time providing clinical services, which could also lead to skills degradation. As we indicated earlier, borrowed military manpower would require a policy be set for the minimum amount of time that the health care professional was required to spend performing clinical duties. In addition, when a CSH is deployed, it would pull many health care professionals from a single MTF, which could result in a substantially reduced ability to deliver the full spectrum of services to the remaining soldiers on base and their dependents. This would limit access to care and potentially affect the quality of care delivered in the MTF.

Reduce Impact of Deployment on Military Treatment Facilities

We heard in our interviews that deployments of PROFIS personnel negatively affect MTFs, and this was supported by our survey results (Figure 4.15). We did not, however, measure the effects of MTF personnel deployments on beneficiary access to care or the workload of remaining MTF personnel using data on workload, productivity, or ability for people to make appointments from MTFs. We describe two modifications to potentially minimize the impact of PROFIS deployments on MTFs: increase civilian staff at the MTFs and develop a national backfill contract for MEDCOM (Table 5.5).

Increase Civilian Staff at Military Treatment Facilities

Some MTFs we visited have already hired more civilian staff. They have recognized that, in the current operating environment, they will always have a certain number of Army health care personnel deployed, so they have tried to increase the number of civilian staff to reduce the strain caused by these deployments. All MTFs should consider this option. However, it will likely be feasible only in cases where there are enough health care professionals in a given specialty in which at least one is almost always deployed. In addition, MTF management need to consider what they will do with these civilian personnel once the current engagements end and military deployments decrease.

Table 5.5
Assessment of Potential Modifications to Reduce Impact of Deployments on MTFs

Potential Modification	Health Care Professional	MTF	Regional Medical Command	AMEDD Leadership	Receiving Unit
Increase civilian staff at MTFs.	Improves	Improves	Improves	Neutral	Neutral
Implement a national backfill contract for regional medical commands/MTFs.	Improves/ neutral	Improves	Improves	Worsens	Neutral

Implement a National Backfill Contract

Many of the staff at the MTFs and regional medical commands we interviewed noted that getting backfill has become increasingly difficult, and, at best, they receive backfill for only one out of every two health care professionals who deploy. Backfill is important because some Army bases are located in areas without robust civilian networks to which patients could be referred, and ten are actually in federally designated primary care health professional shortage areas (e.g., Fort Polk, Fort Irwin). The reserve component does not provide backfill anymore in almost all cases, because of their own deployments and dwell time requirements for reservists. However, our interviewees also noted that developing the actual contracts necessary for hiring civilian professionals to backfill can be difficult. It was suggested that MEDCOM develop a national backfill contracting mechanism, so that each regional medical command or MTF does not have to develop these contracts independently. The Dental and the Nurse Corps already have national backfill contracts. This would mean more work for AMEDD leadership, but might alleviate the problem for MTFs and regional medical commands. It could improve the situation for MTFs if the backfill rates improved.

Reduce Skills Degradation

We describe two potential ways to improve the issue around reported skills degradation: restrict deployments following completion of training and perform more formal reassessments of returning PROFIS professionals (Table 5.6).

Have No Deployment in the Year Following Clinical Training

Currently, some corps and some AOCs within corps attempt to restrict the deployment of personnel immediately after residency, fellowship, or other major training. However, we also observed some trainees being assigned to PROFIS slots while they were still in training, including physician residency programs, knowing that the unit would be deploying within weeks of the completion of that person's training. We believe limiting deployment for a year following training would cause additional stress to the current situation for a year or so because some AOCs and consultants count on newly trained health care professionals to fill PROFIS slots, but that it might not cause significant longer-term stresses, if health care professionals still complete the same number of deployments in their career. Allowing all health care professionals to practice outside of the training environment might allow them to solidify their skills (e.g., allowing a pediatrician to practice as a pediatrician for a year before deploying in a

Table 5.6
Assessment of Potential Modifications to Reduce Skills Degradation During Deployment

Potential Modification	Health Care Professional	MTF	Regional Medical Command	AMEDD Leadership	Receiving Unit
No deployment in year following clinical training (to allow skills to solidify before deployments).	Improves	Improves	Neutral	Improves	Improves
Formal assessment of need for retraining upon redeployment.	Improves	Improves	Neutral	Improves	Neutral

PROFIS position). This is especially true in specialties where health care professionals might not be using these new specialty-specific skills as frequently, or at all, while deployed.

Make a Formal Assessment of Need for Retraining Upon Redeployment

The other modification would be to more routinely assess the skills of returning health care professionals. This would not prevent the degradation of skills while deployed, but would enable identification when it occurs and facilitate regaining skills as rapidly as possible upon redeployment. This might be more important for some corps and some AOCs than others. Currently, the system requires a returning health care professional to self-identify skill loss and need for retraining, which might not be easy for a highly trained professional. They might not want to admit that they have lost some skills, and they often want to return to work quickly to relieve the extra burden that has been placed on the staff who remained at the MTF. A more routine system to assess individuals' skills would alleviate this and would potentially identify individuals who would benefit from some retraining, time to shadow another provider, or time to ease into more complicated clinical activities after returning from deployment.

Improve Other Equity Issues

We identified two other modifications that could improve equity issues (Table 5.7): eliminate the 90-day post stabilization period for some deployers and switch all AOCs to be managed centrally, as Tier I.

Eliminate 90-Day Post-Stabilization Period

This modification suggests eliminating the 90-day post-stabilization period for personnel deployed in a 62B position (most often battalion surgeons) and behavioral health officers (67D). As most PROFIS personnel are deployed with a unit that is not based at their permanent duty station, this is an extra three months away from their families. During our interviews with both FORSCOM and MEDCOM personnel, we heard uncertainty over whether there is a benefit associated with the 90-day post-stabilization period. The benefit should be measured in light of the other resources on base for returning soldiers to use if they need behavioral health services and the fact that some soldiers may prefer to see providers who do not know them and can continue to provide the care they need after 90 days. Since the 90-day redeployment period is a burden to the PROFIS professionals who have deployed, this policy should be thoroughly evaluated.

Table 5.7
Assessment of Other Potential Modifications to Improve Equity of Deployments

Potential Modification	Provider	MTF	Regional Medical Command	AMEDD Leadership	Receiving Unit
Eliminate 90-day post-stabilization period for 62B and behavioral health specialties.	Improves	Improves	Improves	Improves	Neutral
Switch all officer AOCs to Tier I and manage centrally.	Improves	Worsens	Worsens	Worsens	Neutral

Switch All Officer AOCs to Tier I and Manage Centrally

MEDCOM Health Policy and Services tries to fairly distribute Tier II and Tier III PROFIS requirements to the regional medical commands based on assigned strength within each AOC. However, this does not take into account how many personnel might have a permanent or temporary profile, nor does it take into account how many people might be in nondeployable positions or might be fenced by the regional medical command. One solution to this is to switch all officer AOCs to Tier I and manage them centrally by MEDCOM. This might also have the advantage of more evenly distributing requirements from primary AOCs to allowed substitution AOCs to improve the distribution of deployments across different AOCs. However, this would likely significantly increase the workload on MEDCOM Health Policy and Services and human resources operations branch personnel. It would also be difficult for the consultants in large AOCs. MTFs and regional medical commands would lose some control in this process, but it could improve the system for health care professionals if it improved equity of deployments.

Summary

We have presented 23 potential modifications to PROFIS. No one modification addresses all of the issues that stakeholders have regarding PROFIS. And some modifications might make the situation worse for some stakeholders. Our qualitative analysis focused on the five issues identified early in the study: equity, predictability, retention, skills and training, and impact on the MTFs. However, there are other impacts that many of these changes could have, including cost and size of the military or civilian force structure for AMEDD. In the next chapter, we present the options we think are most promising. For each of these options, we describe some of the next steps that might be undertaken as part of a more detailed assessment, which we recommend being performed before any implementation.

CHAPTER SIX

Conclusions and Recommendations

This chapter presents our conclusions and recommendations. Using the information from our analysis of reports about PROFIS and MEDCOM deployments, interviews of Army personnel in AMEED and FORSCOM involved in different aspects of PROFIS, a survey of health care professionals across seven corps in MEDCOM, and analysis of personnel data and PROFIS data on deployments, we arrived at the conclusions listed below:

- PROFIS generally works. It enables the Army to deploy the required number of health care professionals with the appropriate skills, but there are areas for improvement.
- PROFIS is largely viewed as equitable, but a sizable minority view it as inequitable.
- Those who perceive it as inequitable belong to the more frequently deployed skill groups.
- Deployments differ substantially in number and length, depending on the AOC of the health care professional.
- Filling the battalion surgeon position imposes additional demands on some physicians because these positions can include extended deployments and there is more often a skills mismatch.
- Notification of deployment and delivery of formal orders occurs very late in the process for a substantial percentage of PROFIS deployers.
- The PROFIS selection process involves noticeable turmoil that results in negative outcomes for the PROFIS deployers and the units to which they are assigned.
- Some health care professionals report that certain clinical skills degrade during deployment; however, leadership skills are almost universally seen as improving.
- Medical personnel perceive that PROFIS deployments result in increased workload and reduced access to medical care at the MTF from which health care professionals on PROFIS tours deploy.
- Long or multiple deployments and a perception of inequity are associated with decreased propensity of physicians to remain in the military.

Recommendations

While analysis of our data makes it clear that PROFIS generally works, aspects of the program require the attention of senior policymakers. Even if some of the problems are only perceptual, perception equates to reality for the perceiver and can have important consequences.

What we suggest are modifications to a program that works reasonably well. In Chapter Five, we described an array of potential modifications to PROFIS and our qualitative assessment of how the potential modifications would affect different stakeholders. In this section, we identify 11 modifications we view as most promising based on the qualitative assessment and describe preliminary next steps that should be undertaken to further assess these modifications. We note that PROFIS is a relatively complex system and, while each suggested modification improves one aspect of PROFIS, no single modification resolves all issues. Thus, multiple modifications will likely be the best solution for improving PROFIS.

We divide our recommended modifications into two categories. One category contains modifications that we believe can be implemented by themselves and would have an immediate but modest effect. The second category involves modifications that would require an integrated approach but could have substantially greater effect.

We recognize that some suggestions have both upsides and downsides. The modifications presented here were not subjected to a formal assessment. Therefore, they require additional data and analyses to estimate their impact and potential negative effects prior to implementation to ensure that the positive aspects of a recommendation outweigh any negative ones.

Modifications That Could Be Implemented Individually and in the Near Term

Limit consecutive assignments in nondeployable positions. Individuals occupying some AMEDD positions are precluded from deployment. The problem occurs when an individual moves from one sheltered position to another. We do not know the extent to which this practice occurs; however, some perceive it as occurring. The first step to assess the effect of limiting consecutive assignments in nondeployable positions would be to identify all such positions and which AOCs are able to fill them. The second step would be to determine whether personnel do in fact move from nondeployable to nondeployable position. The third step would be to determine whether a limitation policy would make any difference. While our qualitative assessment suggests this change would improve the equity of deployments, the number of health care professionals that would be affected by this recommendation may be so small that it would have no measurable effect on the number of health care professionals who do not deploy. It should be noted, however, that even if this modification would not change the number of health care professionals who do not deploy, it could improve perceptions of equity, which may be reason enough to implement the modification.

Reduce nondeployable profiles in deployable positions. There are a number of health care professionals who have permanent profiles that limit their ability to deploy. In addition, there are positions that have been deemed, by either policy or practice, as nondeployable. Moving personnel with permanent profiles to positions that are nondeployable could increase the supply of personnel available for deployment. The first step would be to determine how many nondeployable positions there are in each corps by category (location, leadership position, AOC, etc.). In addition, the corps would need to determine how many personnel with permanent profiles there are by AOC. In some cases, such as senior leadership positions, the Army will likely want to fill those positions with the best qualified person, regardless of their profile status. However, for other positions, such as smaller MTFs or remote locations, it might be possible to place personnel with permanent profiles in these nondeployable positions.

Provide short-term sick call and trauma refresher before deployment in 62B Tasking for subspecialists and nonpracticing MDs. A minority (20–30 percent) of subspecialists who deploy as battalion surgeons reported not being well prepared for their clinical duties while deployed, which largely involve routine sick call and trauma treatment. Providers should be given the opportunity to refresh themselves in these skills before deploying. They could take part in unit sick calls or pull rotations in emergency rooms as a way of preparing for deployment. Alternatively, refresher modules focused on sick call and trauma situations could be developed. As a precursor to actually developing refresher modules, the first step would be to identify the key clinical activities the battalion surgeon performs. In order to not place an undue burden on deploying health care professionals who do not need the refresher, it would be important to identify the AOCs for whom training is most needed. The refresher could be made available to other health care professionals on a voluntary basis.

Improve timeliness of cutting orders for PROFIS personnel. Forty-five percent of PROFIS deployers responding to our survey reported receiving their orders less than one month prior to the date they were to deploy. Absence of formal orders can impose substantial hardship on the individual deploying. Personnel typically need a copy of their orders to complete some of the activities necessary prior to deployment, including breaking leases and temporary storing of household goods. When they arrive late, soldiers must cram all predeployment actions into a short period. In our interviews, we heard anecdotal evidence that some bases are more effective than others in the timely cutting of orders for PROFIS deployers. Identifying bases that show the ability to consistently cut orders in a timely fashion would be the first step to determining whether there are best practices that could be adopted by other bases.

Implement an ARFORGEN cycle for PROFIS positions. The ARFORGEN process the Army has implemented for its line units provides a degree of predictability. Predictability was an issue raised in our interviews and surveys. Thus, a similar system might benefit medical personnel. For MEDCOM to adopt the ARFORGEN cycle, AR 601-142 would require revision. In addition, MEDCOM would need to change expectations among FORSCOM leadership about when they would receive the names of their PROFIS fillers.

Implement a more formal reassessment of staff skills upon redeployment. Depending on corps, our surveys uncovered reports of clinical skill degradation among 10 to 50 percent of health care professionals who deployed. We do not know the extent of such degradation or if skills degradation is something some health care professionals simply perceive and worry about. We believe that a more formal determination of the extent of the problem is warranted. This evaluation could take many forms, such as the use of simulations or observation by other providers. Because some AOCs could experience skills degradation while others do not, the evaluation would need to be tailored for specific AOCs. If skills degradation is determined to be a problem, the next step would be to identify what skills are most likely to degrade by AOC. Then a process for reassessment of these skills and determining level of skills refreshment needed could be developed. This could be implemented for PROFIS as well as organically deployed health care professionals.

Implement a national backfill contract for regional medical commands/MTFs. Deploying personnel place perceived additional strain on the MTFs, and backfill, especially within some specialties, is a challenge for many MTFs. Some areas have a relatively sparse health care network and lack the personnel to backfill deploying military personnel. One approach to easing the strain on MTFs of deploying medical personnel is to consider a nationwide backfill contract. A national contract could ease administration burdens on the regional medical commands and MTFs and might enable AMEDD to draw replacement staff nationally. The Nurse and Dental Corps have such contracts, and the effectiveness of these contracts should be assessed. If confirmed, the feasibility of other corps adopting similar contracts should be explored to address the needs at MTFs that suffer a disproportionate workload burden from deployment.

Modifications Potentially Best Implemented as an Integrated Approach

The integrated approach involves two modifications designed to increase the supply of health care professionals available for deployment and one modification that is a change to the battalion surgeon position. The three modifications are as follows:

- Shift AMEDD staffing to increase personnel in AOCs in demand for deployment.
- Shift payback for some Army-trained subspecialists from active duty to long-term civilian contracts in MTFs.
- Fill most PROFIS battalion surgeon positions with physician assistants and nurse practitioners.

Collectively, these modifications are designed to improve the equity of deployments, change the composition of Army health care professionals available for deployments to improve the alignment of the skills and training of health care professionals with deployment needs, reduce the impact of deployment on MTFs, and improve retention of health care professionals.

Shift Army medical personnel requirements to increase personnel in AOCs in demand for deployment. This recommendation resulted from the observation that some AOCs deploy much more frequently than others. In addition, many specialists are being deployed as battalion surgeons; these health care professionals frequently report a degradation of their clinical skills while deployed, which in turn reduces their interest in remaining in the military. While the results of this project suggest that the current distribution of personnel in AOCs could be modified to better match deployment needs, many unknowns remain that need to be addressed prior to implementing any changes. The first step would be to review again the overall requirements for personnel in medical AOCs and compare those with the current distribution of personnel in these AOCs and deployment frequencies. While we examined the types of health care professionals that have been deployed, we did not assess the caseload of health care professionals in the MTFs. The next step that should be undertaken is determining the need for specialists in the MTFs. Only when this information is compiled can informed decisions be made about whether the supply of certain AOCs can be reduced. Obviously, this recommendation would require careful analysis and some time to implement.[1]

Shift payback for some Army-trained subspecialists from active duty to long-term civilian contracts in MTFs. Even if the determination is made that the current supply of infrequently deploying specialists is needed for care for soldiers and their dependents in MTFs, it is possible that they do not need to be active duty health care professionals. This recommendation suggests that the Army consider altering the method of paying back the cost of medical training by allowing personnel trained in subspecialties to opt out of serving on active duty in exchange for a long-term contract with the Army to serve in MTFs when needed. This step could provide the Army with a pool of trained personnel that could be available over a substantial period. The feasibility of this approach would need to be determined.

Fill all PROFIS battalion surgeon positions with physician assistants and nurse practitioners. As indicated in the report, the battalion surgeon position poses some unique challenges. A physician assistant or a nurse practitioner could provide the skills needed to conduct routine sick call and deal initially with traumas. While physician assistants act as battalion

---

[1] Buchanan (1983) develops a mathematical programming method for joint analysis of MTF and readiness medical requirements.

surgeons in garrison, nurse practitioners do not take on this role and are not currently approved substitutes for the battalion surgeon position. Therefore, it needs to be assessed whether using nurse practitioners as battalion surgeons is appropriate, specifically whether their skill set is well matched to the duties performed by battalion surgeons. Because physician assistants are the most frequently deployed AMEDD AOC, using physician assistants as battalion surgeons would require increasing the supply of physician assistants. Deploying nurse practitioners as battalion surgeons could require increasing the supply of nurse practitioners as well. Increasing the supply of physician assistants and nurse practitioners would require a number of actions, including modifying the authorization documents and recruiting and training personnel, to generate the number of physician assistants or nurse practitioners required, and thus this is not a simple recommendation to implement. If the supply of physician assistants and nurse practitioners is increased, a second step would be to determine how the Army would utilize this increased supply within MTFs and clinics when not deployed.

Switch battalion surgeon to organic physician assistant/nurse practitioner positions and use borrowed military manpower. A fourth modification could be combined with the integrated approach. In addition to filling all PROFIS battalion surgeon positions with physician assistants/nurse practitioners, these positions also could be converted to organic physician assistant/nurse practitioner positions and a borrowed military manpower model used. Before implementing such a change, AMEDD would need to first determine requirements for the amount of time that physician assistants and nurse practitioners spend in MTFs/clinics and the types of duties they perform in order to maintain their clinical skills and then work with FORSCOM to write and implement a policy to ensure that health care professionals can meet these requirements.

Summary

PROFIS was implemented to help AMEDD meet its dual mission of providing care to deployed soldiers and soldiers in garrison, their families, and other military beneficiaries. While the system has been taxed over the past ten years of constant deployments, it still meets its primary objective. However, our research has documented deficiencies, and we have described possible modifications that the Army could make to improve the system.

PROFIS Areas of Concentration/Military Occupational Specialties, by PROFIS Tier and Number of Army Personnel in Each, as of December 2009

This appendix presents each of the AOC and MOS codes in their PROFIS tier, which are described in Chapter Two. The tiers are used when managing deployment of PROFIS personnel: Tier I is managed and assigned nationally by the consultants, Tier II is managed by the regional medical commands, and Tier III is generally managed at the MTF level.

Table A.1
Tier I AOCs/MOSs

AOC/ MOS	ASI	Specialty	N in Army as of December 2009, Trainees Included
AMEDD Immaterial			
05A		AMEDD Immaterial	2
Medical Corps			
60A		Operational Medicine (immaterial)	0
60C		Preventive Medicine Officer	105
60D		Occupational Medicine Officer	35
60J		Obstetrician and Gynecologist	228
60K		Urologist	73
60N		Anesthesiologist	163
60W		Psychiatrist	145
61A		Nephrologist	19
61J		General Surgeon	300
61K		Thoracic Surgeon	20
61L		Plastic Surgeon	19
61M		Orthopedic Surgeon	256
61N		Flight Surgeon	50
61W		Peripheral Vascular Surgeon	20
61Z		Neurosurgeon	16

Table A.1—Continued

AOC/ MOS	ASI	Specialty	N in Army as of December 2009, Trainees Included
62A		Emergency Medicine Physician	272
Nurse Corps			
66C	7T	Psychiatric/Mental Health Nurse, Clinical Nurse Specialist	65
66C		Psychiatric/Mental Health Nurse	100
66F		Nurse Anesthetist	177
66H	8A	Medical Surgical Nurse, Critical Care Nursing	462
66H	M5	Medical Surgical Nurse, Emergency Nursing	180
66N		Operational Nursing (immaterial)	1
66P		Family Nurse Practitioner	155
Medical Specialist Corps			
65D		Physician Assistant	807
Dental Corps			
63N		Oral & Maxillofacial Surgeon	98
Medical Service Corps			
67A		Health Services Officer (immaterial)	2,722
67D		Behavioral Science Officer (immaterial)	330
70A	5N	Health Care Administrator, Inspector General	11
70K	9I	Health Services Material Officer, Health Facilities Planner	9
71A		Microbiologist	2
71E	8T	Clinical Laboratory Officer, Blood Banking	4
73A		Social Worker	0
73B		Clinical Psychologist	2
Enlisted Corps			
68P	M5	Radiology Specialist, Nuclear Medicine Specialist	62
68S		Preventive Medicine Specialist	702
68V		Respiratory Specialist	251
68W	M3	Health Care Specialist, Dialysis Specialty	37
68W	M6	Health Care Specialist, Practical/Vocational Nurse	1,486

Table A.2
Tier II AOCs/MOSs

AOC/ MOS	ASI	Specialty	N in Army as of December 2009, Trainees Included
Medical Corps			
60B		Nuclear Medicine Officer	21
60F		Pulmonary Disease/Critical Care Officer	49
60G		Gastroenterologist	58
60H		Cardiologist	77
60L		Dermatologist	94
60M		Allergist, Clinical Immunologist	40
60P		Pediatrician	187
60Q		Pediatric Subspecialist	134
60R		Child Neurologist	11
60S		Ophthalmologist	99
60T		Otolaryngologist	87
60U		Child Psychiatrist	47
60V		Neurologist	54
61B		Medical Oncologist/Hematologist	41
61C		Endocrinologist	19
61D		Rheumatologist	16
61E		Clinical Pharmacologist	8
61F		Internist	312
61G		Infectious Disease Officer	64
61H		Family Medicine	526
61P		Physiatrist	55
61Q		Radiation Oncologist	19
61R		Diagnostic Radiologist	221
61U		Pathologist	121
62B		Field Surgeon	156
Nurse Corps			
66E	8J	Perioperative Nurse, Infection Control	4
66E		Perioperative Nurse	283

Table A.2—Continued

AOC/ MOS	ASI	Specialty	N in Army as of December 2009, Trainees Included
Medical Specialist Corps			
65A		Occupational Therapist	89
65B		Physical Therapist	261
65C		Dietitian	152
Dental Corps			
63A		General Dentist	319
63B		Comprehensive Dentist	217
63D		Periodontist	54
63E		Endodontist	62
63F		Prosthodontist	72
63H		Public Health Dentist	7
63K		Pediatric Dentist	24
63M		Orthodontist	37
63P		Oral Pathologist	13
63R		Executive Dentist	0
Medical Service Corps			
67E		Pharmacist	140
70B		Health Services Administration	16
70D		Health Services Systems Manager	0
70E		Patient Administrator	1
Enlisted Corps			
68D		Operating Room Specialist	958
68W	N9	Health Care Specialist, Physical Therapy Specialist	244

Table A.3
Tier III AOCs/MOSs

AOC/ MOS	ASI	Specialty	N in Army as of December 2009, Trainees Included
Nurse Corps			
66H		Medical-Surgical Nurse	1,791
Veterinary Corps			
64A		Field Veterinary Service Officer	185
64B		Veterinary Preventive Medicine Officer	101
64C		Veterinary Laboratory Animal Medicine Officer	56
64D		Veterinary Pathologist	49
64E		Veterinary Comparative Medicine Officer	33
64F		Veterinary Clinical Medicine Officer	34
64Z		Senior Veterinarian (Immaterial)	0
Medical Service Corps			
67B		Laboratory Sciences Officer (Immaterial)	314
67C		Preventive Medicine Officer (Immaterial)	425
67F		Optometrist	127
67G		Podiatrist	25
67J		Aeromedical Evacuation Officer	293
70A		Health Care Administrator	1
70C		Health Services Comptroller	0
70F		Health Services Human Resources Manager	0
70H		Health Services Plans, Operations, Intelligence, Security, and Training	7
70K		Health Services Materiel Officer	1
71B		Biochemist	7
71E		Clinical Laboratory Officer	6
71F		Research Psychologist	1
72A		Nuclear Medicine Science Officer	2
72B		Entomologist	0
72C		Audiologist	2
72D		Environmental Science & Engineer Officer	3
72E		Sanitary Engineering	0

Table A.3—Continued

AOC/ MOS	ASI	Specialty	N in Army as of December 2009, Trainees Included
Enlisted Corps			
68A		Biomedical Equipment Specialist	799
68E	N5	Dental Specialist, Dental Laboratory	160
68E	X2	Dental Specialist, Preventive Dentistry	213
68E		Dental Specialist	1,185
68G		Patient Administration Specialist	800
68H		Optical Laboratory Specialist	147
68J		Medical Logistics Specialist	1,310
68K		Medical Laboratory Specialist	1,867
68M		Nutrition Care Specialist	399
68P		Radiology Specialist	1,016
68Q		Pharmacy Specialist	670
68R		Veterinary Food Inspection Specialist	1,022
68T		Animal Care Specialist	517
68W	N3	Health Care Specialist, Occupational Therapy	108
68W	P1	Health Care Specialist, Orthopedics	256
68W	P2	Health Care Specialist, Ear, Nose, Throat, and Hearing Readiness	111
68W	P3	Health Care Specialist, Optometry/ Ophthalmology	239
68W		Health Care Specialist	19,693
68X		Mental Health Specialist	686
68Z		Chief Medical NCO	96

AOCs, by Strata, Used in the Survey Sampling and Analyses

We developed strata when deploying our survey to ensure adequate representation of certain AOCs, as described in Chapter Three. This appendix presents the number and titles of each strata and lists which specialties are included in each strata.

Table B.1
Strata for Each Corps

Enlisted Corps – 1 strata

Medical Corps – 8 strata

    Family medicine and substitutes

    Subspecialty, procedure-intensive

    Subspecialty, non-procedure-intensive

    Nondirect patient care

    General surgery

    General surgery substitutes

    Specialty surgery

    Other

Dental Corps – 1 strata

Veterinary Corps – 1 strata

Medical Specialist Corps – 1 strata

Nurse Corps – 1 strata

Medical Service Corps – 2 strata

    Behavioral health specialists

    Other specialists

Table B.2
Specific AOCs/MOSs Within Each Strata

AOC/MOS	Specialty
Enlisted Corps	
68A	Biomedical Equipment Specialist
68D	Operating Room Specialist
68E	Dental Specialist
68G	Patient Administration Specialist
68H	Optical Laboratory Specialist
68J	Medical Logistics Specialist
68K	Medical Laboratory Specialist
68M	Nutrition Care Specialist
68P	Radiology Specialist
68Q	Pharmacy Specialist
68R	Veterinary Food Inspection Specialist
68T	Animal Care Specialist
68P	Radiology Specialist
68S	Preventive Medicine Specialist
68V	Respiratory Specialist
68W	Health Care Specialist
68X	Mental Health Specialist
68Z	Chief Medical NCO
Medical Corps	
Family Medicine and Approved Substitutions	
60P	Pediatrician
61F	Internist
61H	Family Medicine
61N	Flight Surgeon
62A	Emergency Medicine Physician
62B	Field Surgeon
General Surgery	
61J	General Surgeon
General Surgery Approved Substitutions	
60J	Obstetrician and Gynecologist
60K	Urologist

Table B.2—Continued

AOC/MOS	Specialty
61K	Thoracic Surgeon
61L	Plastic Surgeon
61W	Peripheral Vascular Surgeon
Specialty Surgery	
60S	Ophthalmologist
60T	Otolaryngologist
61M	Orthopedic Surgeon
61Z	Neurosurgeon
Procedure-Intensive Subspecialists	
60G	Gastroenterologist
60H	Cardiologist
60L	Dermatologist
60N	Anesthesiologist
Non-Procedure-Intensive Subspecialists	
60B	Nuclear Medicine Officer
60F	Pulmonary Disease/Critical Care Officer
60M	Allergist, Clinical Immunologist
60Q	Pediatric Subspecialist
60R	Child Neurologist
60U	Child Psychiatrist
60V	Neurologist
60W	Psychiatrist
61A	Nephrologist
61B	Medical Oncologist/Hematologist
61C	Endocrinologist
61D	Rheumatologist
61E	Clinical Pharmacologist
61G	Infectious Disease Officer
61P	Physiatrist
Nondirect Patient Care	
61Q	Radiation Oncologist
61R	Diagnostic Radiologist
61U	Pathologist

Table B.2—Continued

AOC/MOS	Specialty
Other	
60A	Operational Medicine (immaterial)
60C	Preventive Medicine Officer
60D	Occupational Medicine Officer
Dental Corps	
63A	General Dentist
63B	Comprehensive Dentist
63D	Periodontist
63E	Endodontist
63F	Prosthodontist
63H	Public Health Dentist
63K	Pediatric Dentist
63M	Orthodontist
63N	Oral & Maxillofacial Surgeon
63P	Oral Pathologist
63R	Executive Dentist
Veterinary Corps	
64A	Field Veterinary Service Officer
64B	Veterinary Preventive Medicine Officer
64C	Veterinary Laboratory Animal Medicine Officer
64D	Veterinary Pathologist
64E	Veterinary Comparative Medicine Officer
64F	Veterinary Clinical Medicine Officer
64Z	Senior Veterinarian (Immaterial)
Medical Specialist Corps	
65A	Occupational Therapist
65B	Physical Therapist
65C	Dietitian
65D	Physician Assistant
65X	Allied Operations Specialist (Immaterial)
Nurse Corps	
66B	Army Public Health Nurse
66C	Psychiatric/Mental Health Nurse
66E	Perioperative Nurse

Table B.2—Continued

AOC/MOS	Specialty
66F	Nurse Anesthetist
66G	Obstetric and Gynecologic Nurse
66H	Medical Surgical Nurse
66N	Operational Nursing (immaterial)
66P	Family Nurse Practitioner
Medical Service Corps	
Behavioral Health Specialists	
67D	Behavioral Science Officer (immaterial)
73A	Social Worker
73B	Clinical Psychologist
Other Specialists	
67A	Health Services Officer (immaterial)
67B	Laboratory Sciences Officer (Immaterial)
67C	Preventive Medicine Officer (Immaterial)
67F	Optometrist
67G	Podiatrist
67J	Aeromedical Evacuation Officer
70A	Health Care Administrator
70B	Health Services Administration
70C	Health Services Comptroller
70D	Health Services System Manager
70E	Patient Administrator
70F	Health Services Human Resources Manager
70H	Health Services Plans, Operations, Intelligence, Security, and Training
70K	Health Services Material Officer
71A	Microbiologist
71B	Biochemist
71E	Clinical Laboratory Officer
71F	Research Psychologist
72A	Nuclear Medicine Science Officer
72B	Entomologist
72C	Audiologist
72D	Environmental Science and Engineer Officer
72E	Sanitary Engineering

AOCs That Are Allowed Substitutions for the Battalion Surgeon

The battalion surgeon position is not typically filled by a physician with a 62B (field surgeon) AOC. There are three groups of AOCs that can deploy as battalion surgeons. They are presented here.

Table C.1
Allowed Substitutions for Battalion Surgeon Positions

AOC/MOS ASI	Specialty
Substitution Group 1	
60P	Pediatrician (non–fellowship trained)
61F	Internist
61H	Family Medicine
Substitution Group 2	
60C	Preventive Medicine Officer
60D	Occupational Medicine Officer
60F	Pulmonary Disease/Critical Care Officer
60G	Gastroenterologist
60H	Cardiologist
60Q	Pediatric Subspecialist
60V	Neurologist
61C	Endocrinologist
61D	Rheumatologist
61N	Flight Surgeon
61P	Physiatrist
62A	Emergency Physician
Substitution Group 3	
60J	Obstetrician and Gynecologist
60L	Dermatologist
60M	Allergist, Clinical Immunologist
61B	Medical Oncologist/Hematologist
61E	Clinical Pharmacologist

References

Air Force Instruction (AFI) 10-401, *Air Force Operations Planning and Execution*, Washington, D.C.: Department of the Air Force, July 21, 2010.

Air Force Instruction (AFI) 41-106, *Unit Level Management of Medical Readiness Programs*, Washington, D.C.: Department of the Air Force, July 28, 2009.

Air Force Instruction (AFI) 41-106, *Medical Readiness Program Management*, Washington, D.C.: Department of the Air Force, July 1, 2011.

ALARACT—*See* Pentagon Telecommunications Center.

Army Regulation (AR) 40-68, *Clinical Quality Management*, Washington, D.C.: Department of the Army, revised February 26, 2004, revised May 22, 2009.

Army Regulation (AR) 601-142, *Army Medical Department Professional Filler System*, Washington, D.C.: Department of the Army, 1986.

Army Regulation (AR) 601-142, *Army Medical Department Professional Filler System*, Washington, D.C.: Department of the Army, revised 1995.

Army Regulation (AR) 601-142, *Army Medical Department Professional Filler System*, Washington, D.C.: Department of the Army, revised April 9, 2007.

Buchanan, Joan, *A Methodology for Evaluating Air Force Physicians' Peacetime and Wartime Capabilities*, Santa Monica, Calif.: RAND Corporation, N-1990-AF, July 1983. As of October 3, 2012:
http://www.rand.org/pubs/notes/N1990.html

Bureau of Medicine and Surgery Instruction (BUMEDINST) 6440.5C, *Health Services Augmentation Program (HSAP) Procedures Guide*, Washington, D.C.: Department of the Navy, January 24, 2007.

Casey, Jr., George W., "HQDA Active Component (AC) Manning Guidance for Fiscal Year (FY) 2011," Washington, D.C., December 17, 2010. As of January 28, 2013:
http://www.armyg1.army.mil/mp.asp

Central Intelligence Agency, *The World Factbook 2010*, "Military Service Age and Obligation," Washington, D.C.: Central Intelligence Agency, 2010. As of October 3, 2012:
https://www.cia.gov/library/publications/the-world-factbook/fields/2024.html

ChartsBin Statistics Collector Team, "Military Conscription Policy by Country," ChartsBin.com, 2010. As of October 3, 2012:
http://chartsbin.com/view/1887

Coley, Herbert, A., *Physician Redeployment Refresher Training*, Fort Sam Houston, Tex.: Department of the Army, OTSG/MEDCOM Policy Memo 09-078, September 21, 2009.

DA Washington DC//DAMO-AOC// on behalf of the Surgeon General, "ALARACT 108/2004—The 180-day AMEDD PROFIS/IA Rotation Policy," to ALARACT (All Army Activities), Washington, D.C., June 2004.

Druss, Benjamin G., Steven C. Marcus, Mark Olfson, Terri Tanielian, and Harold A. Pincus, "Trends in Care by Non-Physician Clinicians in the United States," *New England Journal of Medicine*, Vol. 348, 2003, pp. 130–137.

Edgar, Erin P., *Physician Retention in the Army Medical Department*, strategy research project, Carlisle, Pa.: U.S. Army War College, March 16, 2009.

Goymerak, Paul, "Re-Engineering Professional Filler System (PROFIS); Road Ahead for Future Changes," white paper, Washington, D.C.: Human Resources Operations Branch, Department of the Army, April 20, 2007.

Hooker, Roderick S., and Linda E. Berlin, "Trends in the Supply of Physician Assistants and Nurse Practitioners in the United States," *Health Affairs*, Vol. 21, No. 5, 2002, pp. 174–181.

Hooker, Roderick S., and Linda F. McCaig, "Use of Physician Assistants and Nurse Practitioners in Primary Care, 1995–1999." *Health Affairs*, Vol. 20, 2001, pp. 231–238.

Hosek, James, and Paco Martorell, *How Have Deployments During the War on Terrorism Affected Reenlistment?* Santa Monica, Calif.: RAND Corporation, MG-873-OSD, 2009. As of October 3, 2012: http://www.rand.org/pubs/monographs/MG873.html

Hosek, James, and Mark E. Totten, *Serving Away from Home: How Deployments Influence Reenlistment*, Santa Monica, Calif.: RAND Corporation, MR-1594-OSD, 2002. As of October 3, 2012: http://www.rand.org/pubs/monograph_reports/MR1594.html

Individual Augmentation (IA) Gram 09, *Global Support Assignment (GSA) Business Rules*, Washington, D.C.: Department of the Navy, October 7, 2010.

Leonard, Robert E., "The Professional Filler System (PROFIS): Recognized Challenges—Recommended Solutions, research paper presented to the U.S. Army Command and General Staff College in partial fulfillment of the requirements for A462 Combat Health Support Seminar, Fort Leavenworth, Kan., 2002.

Malish, Richard G. (LTC), "The United States Army Battalion Surgeon: Frontline Requirement or Relic of a Bygone Era?" master's thesis, U.S. Army Command and General Staff College, 2009.

Malish, Richard G., Gail L. Maxwell, Ross Witters, Lilia Z. Macias-Moriarity, and Roger L. Gelperin, "Perceptions of Frontline Providers on the Appropriate Qualifications for Battalion Level Care in United States Army Ground Maneuver Forces," *Military Medicine*, Vol. 176, No. 12, 2011 pp. 1369–1375.

Medical Annex to Air Force Instruction 10-401, *Prioritization and Sequencing Guidance*, Washington, D.C: Air Force Medical Service, July 21, 2010.

Nolan, David L., "Airborne Tactical Medical Support in Grenada," *Military Medicine*, Vol. 155, No. 3, 1990, pp. 104–111.

Novier, Frank H., *Balancing Medical Readiness: The Dilemma of Caretaker Hospitals*, U. S. Army War College: Carlisle, Pa., 1993.

Organisation for Economic Co-operation and Development, "OECD Health Data 2010," October 2010.

Pentagon Telecommunications Center on behalf of DA Washington DC/DAPE-MPE//, "ALARACT 253/2007—Individual Dwell Time (IDT) Deployment Policy, to ALARACT (All Army Activities)," Washington, D.C., November 2007.

Pentagon Telecommunications Center on behalf of DA Washington DC/DAPE-MPE//, "ALARACT 214/2009 (Corrected Copy) Stop Loss and Deployment Policy Updates, official correspondence to ALARACT (All Army Activities)," Washington, D.C., August 2009.

Pentagon Telecommunications Center on behalf of DA Washington DC//DASG-HSZ//DAMO-DASG, "ALARACT 306/2009 (Addendum to ALARACT 214/2009) Implementation Instructions for Medical Personnel," official correspondence to ALARACT (All Army Activities), Washington, D.C., October 2009.

Pentagon Telecommunications Center on behalf of DA Washington DC//DASG-HSZ//DAMO-DASG, "ALARACT 013/2012 (Corrected Copy) Updated Professional Filler System (PROFIS) Deployment Periods ISO the Army 270-Day Deployment Period Policy," official correspondence to ALARACT (All Army Activities), Washington, D.C., January 2012.

Robinson, A. M., Jr., *Personnel Rotation Policy*, memorandum for Commanders of Navy Medicine East, Navy Medicine West, Navy Medicine National Capital Area, and Navy Medicine Support Command, Washington, D.C.: Department of the Navy, June 24, 2009.

Roy, C. L., C. L. Liang, M. Lund, C. Boyd, J. T. Katz, S. McKean, and J. L. Schnipper, "Implementation of a Physician Assistant/Hospitalist Service in an Academic Medical Center: Impact on Efficacy and Patient Outcomes," *Journal of Hospital Medicine*, Vol. 3, No. 5, 2008, pp. 361–368.

Sarmiento, Don J., "After Action Report: March 2, 2003," Kuwait: 187th Infantry Regiment, 101st Airborne Division. Reprinted in *The Medical Soldiers Outlook: Army Medical Department Enlisted Training News*, Vol. 23, No. 3, Fall 2004.

Schoomaker, Eric B., *PROFIS/IA Replacement Policy for Operation Iraqi and Enduring Freedom*, OTSG/MEDCOM Policy Memo 09-014, Fort Sam Houston, Tex.: Department of the Army, March 18, 2009.

Schoomaker, Eric B., *PROFIS/Individual Augmentee (IA) Replacement policy for Operation Enduring Freedom and Operation New Dawn*, OTSG/MEDCOM Policy Memo 11-024, Fort Sam Houston, Tex.: Department of the Army, March 22, 2011.

Schwartz, Norton A., *Change to Air Expeditionary Force (AEF) Baseline*, memorandum for distribution, Washington, D.C.: Department of the Air Force, September 2, 2010.

Shaeffer, Joseph, ed., *IDO & UDM: Guide to the AEF*, Version 4.0 (FOUO), Randolph AFB, Tex.: Air Force Personnel Center, June 1, 2011.

Sox Jr., Harold C., "Quality of Patient Care by Nurse Practitioners and Physician's Assistants: A Ten-Year Perspective," *Annals of Internal Medicine*, Vol. 91, No. 3, 1979, pp. 459–468.

U.S. Army Medical Command, *PROFIS Handbook*, 3rd ed., January 2011.

War Resisters International, "Sweden," 2009. As of October 3, 2012: http://www.wri-irg.org/programmes/world_survey/reports/Sweden